Health Ess...

Shiatsu

Elaine Liechti was Secretary of the Shiatsu Society UK from its formation in 1981 until 1990. She is a member of the Shiatsu Society's Practitioner Assessment Panel and is Director of the Glasgow School of Shiatsu.

The Health Essentials Series

There is a growing number of people who find themselves attracted to holistic or alternative therapies and natural approaches to maintaining optimum health and vitality. The *Health Essentials* series is designed to help the newcomer by presenting high quality introductions to all the main complementary health subjects. Each book presents all the essential information on each therapy, explaining what it is, how it works and what it can do for the reader. Advice is also given, where possible, on how to begin using the therapy at home, together with comprehensive lists of courses and classes available worldwide.

The *Health Essentials* titles are all written by practising experts in their fields. Exceptionally clear and concise, each text is supported by attractive illustrations.

Series Medical Consultant
Dr John Cosh MD, FRCP

In the same series

Alexander Technique by Richard Brennan
Aromatherapy by Christine Wildwood
Flower Remedies by Christine Wildwood
Reflexology by Inge Dougans with Suzanne Ellis
Spiritual Healing by Jack Angelo

Health Essentials

SHIATSU

Japanese Massage for Health and Fitness

ELAINE LIECHTI

ELEMENT
Shaftesbury, Dorset ● Rockport, Massachusetts

© Elaine Liechti 1992

Published in Great Britain in 1992 by
Element Books Limited
Longmead, Shaftesbury, Dorset

Published in the USA in 1992 by
Element, Inc
42 Broadway, Rockport, MA 01966

Cover illustration from an Eric Gill woodcut
Cover design by Max Fairbrother
Illustrations by David Gifford
Diagrams by Taurus Graphics
Typeset by Falcon Typographic Art Ltd, Edinburgh
Printed and bound in Great Britain by
Billings Ltd, Hylton Road, Worcester

A catalogue record for this book
is available from the British Library

Library of Congress Data available

ISBN 1–85230–318–2

Note from the Publisher
Any information given in any book in the *Health Essentials* series is
not intended to be taken as a replacement for medical advice. Any
person with a condition requiring medical attention should consult
a qualified medical practitioner or suitable therapist.

Contents

To all my teachers, my patients, and especially my students who are a constant source of learning and inspiration. To my parents for their encouragement, and most of all to my husband John and my daughter Cora for their love and support.

1

What is Shiatsu?

SHIATSU AS THERAPY

S HIATSU IS A healing art, originating in Japan, which uses the
power of touch and pressure to enable each of us to contact
our own self-healing abilities. In a Shiatsu session the practitioner
uses pressure with thumbs, fingers, palms, and sometimes elbows,
knees and feet, to induce deep relaxation and a feeling of
well-being. It is sometimes a dynamic, sometimes a seemingly
static form, involving pressure and stretching on the limbs and
torso, kneading and releasing tight muscles, and supporting
areas of weakness. To receive, Shiatsu is deeply relaxing and
yet invigorating, leaving a feeling of tranquillity and a sense of
being in touch with every part of one's body. Giving Shiatsu is
like performing a moving meditation and leaves the giver feeling
as balanced and energized as the receiver.

Shiatsu was developed from traditional oriental massage
and, in common with acupuncture and other oriental therapies, it works upon the body's energetic system, using the
network of meridians or energy pathways which relates to the
functioning of the internal organs as well as our emotional,
psychological and spiritual harmony. The concept of the
body as an 'energetic' organism comes from ancient Chinese
thought, and through centuries of experience and study has
evolved into a system of medical theory which is both rich
and poetic. Energy, known as *Ki* in Japanese (*Qi* in Chinese),
flows throughout the body, rather like a system of rivers

1

and canals. Things may happen to upset the smooth flow of Ki causing blockages or dams in some areas, weaknesses or stagnant pools in others. These in turn may lead to physical symptoms, psychological or emotional disturbance, or a feeling that 'things are just not quite right'.

Shiatsu uses physical pressure and meridian stretches to unblock the dams – which show up as tight muscles and areas of stiffness – and revitalize the empty areas – which may feel cold, weak or just needing to be held. Oriental medical theory provides a framework by which the practitioner can assess the body's energetic state and needs, and can explain why the body holds tension in certain areas or points and feels weak in others.

THE POWER OF TOUCH

The techniques used in Shiatsu are both simple and profound. We are all familiar with 'the healing power of touch'. Every mother knows that a kiss and 'let Mummy rub it better' is more effective than Elastoplast; athletes find that immediate local massage can do much to restore a pulled muscle, and who has not felt better for a cuddle in times of emotional stress? Yet although we are aware at a common-sense level that we need touch, our society has largely educated that intuitive feeling out of us, so that it is not socially acceptable to ask for or give physical contact unless in an extreme or traumatic situation.

All forms of bodywork and massage can fulfill the need for touch, but Shiatsu is particularly applicable and practical in an everyday setting for a variety of reasons. One important aspect is that the receiver remains clothed during the treatment. In a society where we have inhibitions about being touched, removing clothes is a further challenge that can leave the receiver feeling uncomfortably vulnerable. Secondly, the slow and sustained holding pressure which characterizes Shiatsu actively encourages conscious relaxation. This allows the physiological mechanisms governing muscle tension to release more efficiently than with some other forms of bodywork. Thirdly, Shiatsu is very practical: it requires no special equipment, just a blanket or mat on the floor, and peace and quiet. And fourthly, although Shiatsu can be used to treat a number of serious complaints when practised by a fully trained therapist, the basics can be mastered by anyone taking introductory classes. The knowledge gained at this level is sufficient to ease everyday aches, pains and minor problems in a family or work setting or between friends. Indeed this is possibly one of the greatest strengths of Shiatsu. In Japan, Shiatsu is widely used as a home remedy. In this context it can do a great deal to strengthen human relationships and provide compassionate support in times of trouble.

PREVENTION AND TREATMENT OF ILLNESS

Like other natural healing and alternative therapies, Shiatsu is concerned with preventative measures. Shiatsu keeps the body healthy, flexible and in balance, as well as monitoring the energetic changes that may be precursors of sickness. In the oriental view, an imbalance of Ki develops before the symptoms of illness occur. Regular Shiatsu treatment can help to pinpoint any patterns of imbalance in the body's Ki structure by ironing out those disturbances before they become entrenched. In the case of people already suffering from health problems, Shiatsu can be of great benefit, both as a discipline in its own right and in concert with other complementary and orthodox treatments. Many conditions are particularly suitable for Shiatsu treatment, including headaches and migraine, acute and chronic back pain (especially if of muscular origin), sciatica, muscular stiffness and injuries, some forms of arthritis and rheumatic complaints. Working as it does on the body's internal organs, Shiatsu can also have a role in the treatment of digestive and intestinal disorders, circulatory, respiratory and reproductive problems. Because Shiatsu works on relaxing the body at a deep level and contacting the more subtle aspects of one's energetic make-up, it can also help in the treatment of anxiety, tension, depression and emotional instability.

An experienced Shiatsu practitioner may explain the imbalance in terms of oriental theory to help the patient understand their own condition. Some practitioners suggest dietary and lifestyle changes to aid healing. Stretching exercises and points to press may form part of a patient's 'homework' to sustain the effect of the treatment between sessions.

THE SESSION ITSELF

The format of a Shiatsu session will vary according to the degree of experience and expertise of the practitioner. Beginners tend to follow a 'form' in which all the meridians are generally stimulated, producing an overall relaxing effect. An experienced professional practitioner generally only begins a series of treatments after taking a detailed case history from the patient. By palpating the abdomen (known in Japanese as the *hara*) and the back, and possibly by feeling the pulses, the patient's energetic state can be assessed. From the information gained, the practitioner may choose to work on one, two, or more meridians, using stretches to open the body before stimulating the points. The techniques used depend entirely upon the patient's energetic state and needs. More dynamic moves such as rocking, shaking and stretching help to disperse and move blocked Ki. Long, deep thumb pressure on specific points or palming a meridian helps to draw Ki to areas of weakness and emptiness. When working on large or heavily muscled people the practitioner may make extensive use of elbows, knees and feet. This is in order to be more effective in contacting the Ki. It also prevents the practitioner from becoming over-tired when moving a large body about. When working on children, babies or very elderly patients, pressure is usually very light, and some practitioners even work at the etheric level, that is, above the body but within the body's energetic field, where physical pressure is inappropriate.

No two Shiatsu sessions are ever alike. The order of work, the choice of meridians to be stimulated and the areas on which to concentrate always change with the receiver's condition. This makes Shiatsu stimulating to give as well as to receive. Here the practitioner's creativity comes into play, blending intuition and knowledge of theory in order to construct a complete and appropriate session for that patient at that time. So each Shiatsu session is a unique event.

Within each session there is a balance between general work, with mobilization and stretches, and specific work on certain meridians. By concentrating on a particular meridian and its associated functions, the practitioner can focus the receiver's self-healing abilities where they are most needed to get to the heart of the problem – an important point when working on someone with very low energy.

Unlike acupuncture or acupressure massage, where the therapist concentrates on a few specific points, in Shiatsu the whole of an imbalanced meridian (or long stretches of it), are stimulated. There is an emphasis on normalizing the muscles and joints around the meridian as well as regulating the Ki in that particular channel. While making use of the traditional acupuncture points, known in Japanese as *tsubo*, Shiatsu also recognizes that Ki may be disturbed anywhere along a meridian. Practitioners therefore work all along the meridians using intuition and developed sensitivity in the hands to locate imbalanced points and bring their energy to the same level as the rest of the meridian. Very often this involves long and slow holding with the degree of pressure depending on the feel of the tsubo. This holding of points is characteristic to Shiatsu, often making it look as though nothing is happening in the treatment. However, the patient will have an intense consciousness of being connected to that point, while at a physiological level the static pressure allows chronically tight muscles to release. Since emotions, old thoughts and memories can be locked up in the soft tissues of the body, Shiatsu practitioners often find that patients experience emotional release during treatment. In the long term this can help deep-seated psycho-emotional conditions.

During the session the practitioner generally works all over the body: arms, legs, back, abdomen, neck and head. This overall treatment again gives the patient the sense of being put back in touch with the whole body, not just the part that may be the current problem. Connecting up the parts draws attention to the relationships between parts of the physical body and the mind.

THE EFFECTS OF TREATMENT

At the end of the treatment the patient is left to rest for a little while. In fact people often fall asleep during the session so a few minutes of recovery time are therefore essential before 'coming back to the here and now'. After treatment the patient usually feels very relaxed, with a sense of well-being and peace.

Sometimes there is also a feeling of invigoration, increased 'get up and go'. Both of these reactions can be put down to the deep energetic effect of the work. Occasionally a new patient may have a 'healing reaction' after a first session. This occurs when toxins have been released during the treatment, and as these work out through the body there may be symptoms such as headache, stiffness, stomach upset or diarrhoea, desire to urinate frequently, or lethargy. Such symptoms are transitory and soon pass, usually in twelve hours at most, although an emotional release may take longer to work through. Drinking plenty of spring water and resting will help, as well as asking the practitioner for advice and reassurance if you are at all worried.

While working meridians and specific points helps to regulate the energetic level, pressure also has the physical effect of stimulating the circulatory, lymphatic and hormonal systems, as well as regulating the activity of both divisions of the autonomic nervous system and releasing toxins.

These all help to activate the body's self-healing mechanisms. Shiatsu practitioners acknowledge that the healing which takes place during a session is largely due to the stimulation of the patient's self-healing abilities. The practitioner is seen as a catalyst who draws attention to certain aspects of the body, mind or spirit which are not functioning properly. It is not uncommon for patients to say after a session: 'I didn't know that that point hurt (was tight, or needed to be touched) until you pressed it.' We are so often 'out of touch' with our bodies and our needs; the caring and compassionate contact between practitioner and patient in Shiatsu can do much to reintroduce ourselves to our bodies and in so doing can help to ease any feelings of alienation and lack of communication with others.

PRACTICALITIES

Shiatsu is very practical in that very little equipment is required. It is almost always practised on the floor, on a thin Japanese cotton futon or mattress. This practice has arisen through tradition; in Japan there is very little space in dwellings and people sleep on futons which can be rolled up during the day leaving the living space clear. However, there are other practical considerations: being at floor level means the practitioner can use body weight rather than muscle power to apply pressure. This is much more comfortable to receive, and certainly less tiring on the practitioner. Shiatsu can also be given in a sitting position on a chair, or lying on the side – useful for pregnant women and people with certain back or chest conditions. All these factors make it very easy to give Shiatsu wherever you are; at home, in the office, even on the beach! Of course professional treatment with a qualified practitioner takes place in a more formal treatment room, which is light, airy and comfortably warm. Some practitioners go out of their way to create a harmonious atmosphere in the room, so that the session is a complete experience involving all five senses, rather like experiencing a Japanese tea ceremony.

Shiatsu is performed through light clothing – a cotton track suit or similar garment is ideal to keep the receiver warm since Shiatsu tends to slow the metabolic rate which can lead to a feeling of coldness. Paradoxically, working through clothes enables the practitioner to concentrate on the feel of the tsubos rather than being distracted by looking. It is interesting to note that in Japan Shiatsu is one of the recognized professions for the blind, whose sense of touch can be so finely developed.

It is usually recommended that patients should not take alcohol or especially large meals on the day of treatment. Lingering in a hot bath and more than normal exercise should also be avoided since all of these tend to disturb the body's Ki and so detract from the effect of the treatment.

SHIATSU AND OTHER THERAPIES

Where does Shiatsu stand in relation to other therapies? I feel that Shiatsu occupies an area of middle ground between acupuncture, massage and healing, as it shares certain essential aspects with each of these disciplines. The combination of these forms a unique and powerful tool for healing and change. Shiatsu has a very distinctive feel which is unlike other forms of bodywork, and this often comes as a surprise to people accustomed to experiencing massage, aromatherapy or reflexology.

Let us look at the common elements and the differences between Shiatsu, Massage, Healing and Acupuncture.

Massage

Massage and Shiatsu share many aspects: the warm and compassionate touch of another human being, encouraging the body to let go and relax. Both forms work on the physical site of pain or stiffness and can release emotional disturbances. Western massage theory and a knowledge of physiology can be used to explain the mechanisms of physical dysfunction. Shiatsu, on the other hand, also enjoys the more poetic yet commonsense explanation embodied in oriental medical theory to give the patient an overall view of the condition. Where Shiatsu differs from most forms of massage, apart from the obvious aspects mentioned earlier, such as being performed through clothing, is in its use of manipulation and stretches.

By manipulation I do not necessarily mean the adjustment of bones, as in osteopathy or chiropractic, although some practitioners do routinely use these techniques. Manipulation in Shiatsu is the use of passive rotations and stretches. For example, picking up the knee and lower leg of a patient lying face upwards and making a wide circle to mobilize and stretch the hip joint. This is a standard physiotherapy technique and one which is widely used in Shiatsu as it gives a good guide to the general overall level of relaxation of the patient. The 'helpful' patient who cannot relax sufficiently to allow the practitioner to do the rotation is often the sort of person who cannot 'let go' in other aspects of life. How wide a circle can the knee make? This indicates overall flexibility. Are there any directions or parts of the rotation that are more difficult or uncomfortable? Each direction or sector of the circle relates to a different meridian function and so a rotation can actually be used as a diagnostic tool to back up other observations about the patient's state.

Rotations are used on shoulders, wrists, ankles, fingers and toes, and gently on the neck. Some practitioners use specific adjustment techniques where they feel there is a need. This is usually effected by putting the receiver into a stretch position and encouraging them to breath through an extension of the stretch. Specific stretches are used to activate a particular area covered by a meridian making it easier to contact and its Ki more open to change.

Anyone who has practised yoga will be aware of the different effects of stretching various parts of the body. This can open up the internal organs and the limbs, bringing about a sense of more flow and vitality. Shiatsu works on the same basis; that by opening the body into a comfortably sustainable stretch, the body's Ki flow can be enhanced and the pressure work made more effective.

Most forms of massage involve the use of oils and moving over the body's surface. Obviously the depth of the massage depends upon the form and the particular practitioner. Some forms of aromatherapy and lymphatic drainage use a very light touch, while Rolfing and Postural Integration work very deeply on the fascia and connective tissues. In Shiatsu we have a contrasting static holding pressure which feels less 'busy'. It fits in very well with the Zen aspect of the therapy (there is a specific form of Shiatsu known as Zen Shiatsu) by concentrating on one point 'right here, right now'. Perhaps it is this stillness which gives Shiatsu its peaceful sense, which is often the overriding sensation after a session. One may feel that a lot of work has been done, pressures released, pain eased, relaxation gained, yet there is tranquillity and peacefulness.

Healing

Healing, the laying on of hands, has a long and well documented history. It is an ability to bring relief to others in a way that is, at present, beyond the scope of science and intellectual thought to explain. In healing, areas of pain are held, usually lightly, and the practitioner directs healing energy, often in the form of light or colour, to the affected area. The patient often has a sensation of warmth, movement or a breeze passing by the part being worked upon. Knowing where to place the hands and when to move to another area depends upon intuition and experience. Most of us have had our intuition educated out of us, and it takes time to learn to listen to and trust the small still voice that says 'work on the right side of the neck' or 'hold the liver area'.

In Shiatsu we have oriental medical theory on which to base

9

what we do, but we can make extensive use of the techniques of healing. Often just holding a point or area and visualizing healing energy entering can be the most powerful part of a treatment, although to the onlooker it would seem as though nothing was happening. These techniques are taught quite early on to students beginning Shiatsu and may account for the reason that beginners often have spectacular successes dealing with common ailments, with little or no knowledge of theory.

Some healers are members of religious organizations and feel that their 'gift' comes from God. Others develop their healing skills through meditation, yoga and other activities. Most have a belief that healing comes not from the practitioner, but through him or her from some much larger entity, call it God, Spirit, Universe, whatever feels appropriate. It is my belief that everyone has the ability to heal – some people just discover it sooner than others and choose to develop it. I would say that everyone in the 'caring professions', orthodox or alternative, is there because of their desire and ability to heal others. Technique is the framework on which to hang the cloth of intuitive healing ability. The choice of technique or discipline depends upon the individual. Personally I chose Shiatsu because it allows me to be very intuitive and creative, yet has a firm theoretical basis which my mind can get to grips with.

Acupuncture

Acupuncture and Shiatsu have common roots and share elements of theory. Whether a patient chooses acupuncture or Shiatsu as a therapy will depend upon personal preference, and upon the health condition. Some people like the physical closeness of Shiatsu with its nurturing and cosseting feeling. Others like the distance of the needles. Practitioners who use both techniques tend to use acupuncture for acute, painful conditions such as arthritis, migraine, frozen shoulder and any kind of blockage or pain. They see Shiatsu as a more nourishing and tonifying therapy which works well for chronic persistent conditions which need long work at a deeper level. Therapists who use both techniques might use acupuncture for the first part of a session to relieve acute pain and increase mobility;

Shiatsu would then be used to rebalance the underlying condition, which is often due to a lack of Ki energy in certain meridians and points. Shiatsu tends to be closer in technique to Japanese acupuncture than to Chinese acupuncture (which is most widely practised in Britain).

One of the basic differences between the two disciplines is in diagnosis. In Shiatsu, because touch is involved in both the diagnosis and the work, we say that diagnosis and treatment are the same. That is,, the practitioner is constantly diagnosing thoughout the treatment, reassessing what he is feeling and modifying the session accordingly. Diagnosis is a fusion of the intuitive feelings which one gains from working on the body, and the intellectual knowledge of theory.

In acupuncture the process is very different and much more intellectually based. The acupuncturist takes the pulses, and then decides upon a principle of treatment, choosing a formulae of points which will have the specific actions needed to remedy the condition. It is rare for the treatment plan to change once the principle and points have been selected.

Japanese acupuncture tends to be more intuitive. A general principle of treatment is to find the most *kyo* or deficient points and tonify them. This may involve the use of the *Theory of Five Elements* to tone up certain points, or it may involve palpating each meridian and quickly needling each deficient point. It is interesting to note that in Japan all acupuncturists learn Shiatsu as part of their training. It is used as a medium for teaching Acupuncture, helping students to 'get in touch with the Ki'.

Perhaps the difference between Shiatsu and acupuncture could be summarized by saying that Shiatsu works physically on the whole body by stimulating Ki along the length of the meridians. The acupuncturist, on the other hand, looks at the whole body and then using the theory of action of points decides which recipe of points will most affect the whole. To quote a patient, Shiatsu gives the feeling of 'being done all over'.

To my mind it is one of the strengths of Shiatsu that it shares elements with other disciplines and integrates them into a unique whole. Theory and manipulation of Ki from the oriental tradition; physiology and some technique from western massage; intuition and openness to universal power from healing. Shiatsu is also very compatible with other therapies and with orthodox medical treatment. It is common for practitioners to use Shiatsu in combination with, say, herbalism, dietary therapy or counselling. Using more than one therapeutic approach can back up the Shiatsu and allow the patient to work through their condition on several different levels at once. Medical practitioners are becoming more familiar with the concepts of alternative and complementary medicine, and it is not unusual for a patient to remark that they checked with their doctor who was quite happy for them to have Shiatsu treatment. As a teacher of Shiatsu, I find a lot of nurses and physiotherapists wish to learn Shiatsu, and those who train to intermediate level and beyond find that they can integrate the new knowledge into their existing work, often with excellent results.

SHIATSU AS SELF DEVELOPMENT

One of the elements of Shiatsu not often discussed in books is the self development aspect. Shiatsu is not just a technique, to be applied during practice hours only and left behind on leaving work for the day. To *be* a Shiatsu practitioner you must take the principles and theory into your heart so that Shiatsu becomes part of every aspect of your life. In the same way that yoga, meditation or the martial arts can be a mirror in which progress through life is seen, so Shiatsu can become the focal point by which your relationship with Self, with others and with life is measured. When the Shiatsu is going well, diagnosis becomes very clear and easy, techniques flow smoothly, intuitive feelings become certainties and the appropriate things are said and done to promote healing. In short, good Shiatsu feels as good to give as to receive.

Students of Shiatsu often begin as patients and, finding that Shiatsu can provide a framework for self understanding, embark upon the study of Shiatsu as a voyage of further self-discovery. The helping and healing of others through the technique of Shiatsu is almost, in a sense, a by-product of the process of self development. The ability to help and heal is in direct ratio to the amount of personal work the student is prepared to put in. A practitioner of Shiatsu cannot be really effective if his or her energetic state is still not balanced and harmonious. Knowing theory and technique alone is not sufficient; the Ki must be strong, and this leads to a healthy body and well balanced outlook on life.

It is not unusual for students to experience big changes in their lives during the course of their study. As their perception of the world changes with their new knowledge and new sensitivity to energy, so personal issues often come forwards to be dealt with. These may be in terms of relationships, reappraising one's work or aim in life, dealing with bereavement or birth, healing a longstanding illness. Within the 'safe' setting of the Shiatsu class, problems can be discussed, support given and, using the principles of Shiatsu, treatment to help the individual through the experience can be worked out. Students are encouraged to look at themselves in depth and work on their own health, physically, emotionally and spiritually.

Self development is implicit in the teaching of Shiatsu. Classes usually begin with a period of Do-in (self Shiatsu), stretching, Qi Gong exercises (similar to Tai Chi) or a general warming up routine. This may be followed by meditation, breathing exercises or Ki sensitivity exercises to develop the students' awareness of Ki. This discipline, begun in class, extends into the life of the practitioner. Most practise meditation, yoga or Shiatsu-related stretching as part of the daily routine, ensuring physical fitness and psychological well being. And of course the practice of Shiatsu itself brings into play the practitioner's own Ki flow. By deep breathing and by applying Ki to the patient, the practitioner's Ki is mobilized, thus stimulating the patient's Ki to flow where it is most needed. When the practitioner's Ki quality is weak or disturbed, this will affect the quality of Shiatsu given; likewise when the Ki is strong, and the practitioner is 'on form', the ability to stimulate the patient's Ki and promote healing is enhanced.

So we can see that Shiatsu is a two-way process. The practitioner lends skill, experience and knowledge as a catalyst in the patient's self-healing. The patient lends himself as the medium through which the therapist can practise his art. This exchange of energy illustrates one of the prime laws of the universe – that everything is changing and energy is always in a constant state of flow and change.

2

The History of Shiatsu

T O DISCOVER THE historical roots of Shiatsu we must go back to ancient China, where the basic principles of all forms of oriental medicine originated. It must first of all be clearly understood that oriental medical theory arose from, and is part of, Chinese philosophy. In the West we tend to think of medicine as being a distinct discipline, having nothing in common with, for example, politics, philosophy or art. In contrast the theories underpinning oriental medicine are the same as those underpinning Chinese thought, culture, art, religion, philosophy, politics, and so on. In other words the ancient Chinese formulated certain principles which were perceived as universal truths and they applied those principles to the realm of medicine. It is probably this very fact which has ensured the continuation of the practice of oriental medicine in largely the same form for centuries, although it must be said that modern Chinese teaching tends to ignore some of the more esoteric and philosophical aspects.

THE EARLY HISTORY OF ORIENTAL MEDICINE

The very early history of oriental medicine is so old as to be clouded in uncertainty and a degree of myth, but the practice of Acupuncture is known to date from before 2500 BC. A bronze model showing Acupuncture points and meridians has been dated at around AD 860. The oldest existing medical text is the *Huang Ti Nei Ching Su Wen* (usually abbreviated to *Nei Ching*) – *The Yellow Emperor's Classic of Internal Medicine*, said to have been written by Huang Ti, the legendary Yellow Emperor who died about 2598 BC. This work is still a respected and oft-quoted source and is an important area of study in modern acupuncture teaching. There is scholarly debate, however, as to the exact authorship and dating of the work. The earliest mention of the *Nei Ching* is made during the first part of the Han Dynasty (206 BC – AD 25). Later editions and commentaries further cloud the original date and authorship, however, as Ilza Veith states in the introduction to the University of California Press edition of the *Nei Ching*:

> it is fair to assume that a great part of the text existed during the Han dynasty, and that much of it is of considerably older origin, possibly handed down by oral tradition from China's earliest history.
>
> *The Yellow Emperor's Classic of Internal Medicine*

The text is in the form of a dialogue between the Yellow Emperor and his minister Ch'i Po, in which the Emperor asks questions on the subject of health and medicine, and Ch'i Po replies at length drawing upon medical theory and philosophical beliefs.

> This form of writing makes it possible to enlarge the scope of the work far beyond that of a medical textbook and to change it into a treatise on general ethics and regimen of life, and to include in it the prevailing Chinese religious beliefs. This combination is, as a matter of fact, the only way in which early Chinese medical thinking could be expressed, for medicine was but a part of philosophy and religion, both of which propounded oneness with nature, i.e. the universe.
>
> Ibid

The *Nei Ching* makes reference to the geographical factors which affected the early development of medical techniques in China. There were two distinct branches of medicine. The Northern methods, from the Yellow River basin where vegetation was sparse and the climate cold, comprised predominantly acupuncture, moxibustion and massage. The Southern tradition originated in the Yangtze River region where the climate was warmer and there was a variety of abundant plant life enabling the people in this area to use the roots, leaves and bark of plants and other substances to form a very comprehensive system of herbal treatment. Both traditions arose from the climactic and environmental influences of their respective regions and in response to the kinds of illnesses which were common in those areas.

The *Nei Ching* goes into detail about which diseases are found in which area and what is the appropriate form of treatment. It mentions the people of the East whose diet of fish and salt causes them to 'burn within' producing ulcers, which are best treated with flint needle acupuncture. The people of the North are subject to many diseases due to the cold, and moxibustion is the appropriate remedy. Moxibustion is the burning of mugwort over particular points and areas in order to introduce heat and stimulate local circulation. Each area, North, South, East, West and Centre is noted. Massage is the specific treatment for the people of the Central region of China.

> The region of the centre, the Earth, is level and moist. Everything that is created by the Universe meets in the centre and is absorbed by the Earth. The people of the regions of the centre eat mixed food and do not (suffer or weary at their) toil. Their diseases are many: they suffer from complete paralysis and chills and fever. These diseases are most fittingly treated with breathing exercises, massage of the skin and flesh, and exercises of the hands and feet. Hence the treatment with breathing exercises, massage and exercises of the limbs has its origin in the centre regions.
>
> *The Yellow Emperor's Classic of Internal Medicine*

The Northern and Southern methods were brought together to form a comprehensive theory of medicine under the Han Dynasty (206BC – AD 220) when China was unified.

Massage was thus from the very first acknowledged as one of the four classical forms of medical treatment, along with acupuncture, moxibustion and herbalism. The form of massage used was called *Anmo* or *Mo* (or *Anma* in Japan) and employed a combination of rubbing and pressing stiff and sore areas. (Modern Chinese massage is known as Tui Na.) The discovery of which areas and points were effective for which conditions no doubt evolved over centuries of experience, observation and trial and error. This knowledge would have been largely transmitted by word of mouth from doctor to apprentice, mother to daughter and so on. Evidence of this lies in the fact that acupuncture has been well documented from the earliest writings but textbooks on Anmo methods are relatively rare, and often incorporate breathing and movement exercises such as Qi Gong, Tai Chi and Tao Yin. In *The History of Scientific Thought, volume 2*, Joseph Needham writes that Chinese massage (Mo) generated a large body of works, the principal ones being *The Manual of Nourishing the Life by Gymnastics* (date unknown) and *Eight Chapters on putting oneself in accord with the Life Force* by Kao Lien, dated 1591.

There are those who believe that massage using the body's energetic flows actually predates acupuncture. Certainly from a practical point of view it seems to make sense that a system of pressing and rubbing the body with the hands should develop before the use of tools (that is, acupuncture needles). It is also interesting that modern-day acupuncturists are usually taught manual palpation of points and massage in order to familiarize them with the body's energy before they are allowed to use needles. Possible evidence for the theory that acupuncture developed later than massage and moxibustion comes in the relatively recent discovery of a text dated before the *Nei Ching* in which 'No points are mentioned, just entire Meridians, portraying zones of influence needing stimulation by moxibustion. This evidence suggests Meridians existed before points.' (T. Kaptchuk, *Chinese Medicine: The Web that has no Weaver.*) What is meant here is that *knowledge* of meridians and the application of technique to the meridians existed before knowledge of the use of points.

PHILOSOPHICAL INFLUENCES

As noted earlier, the theories essential to the practice of medicine were part of the overall Chinese view of the world, in other words, philosophy. The most inherent and widely known of these are the theories of *Yin Yang* and the *Five Elements*, which spring from the underlying concept of *Tao*. (We shall be looking at the actual theories themselves in depth in Chapter 3.)

The *Tao*, usually translated as the *Way*, is an explanation of how the universe came into being, how the forces at work in the universe interplay, and how people can harmonize with nature by adhering to the Tao. It is easy to understand how the ancient Chinese, who were an agriculture-based society, would have seen the cycles and forces at work in nature and developed a system of beliefs and behaviour which mirrored the processes they observed in nature itself. Proof of someone's adherence to the Tao was said to be seen in their state of health and longevity; many ancient Chinese texts make reference to the sages of times past who had lived for well over a hundred years. The formalization of this philosophy of 'going with the flow' took place with the development of Taoism, and the writing of the *Tao Te Ching* by Lao Tzu around the sixth century BC. However, the concepts of Tao and Yin Yang had been part of the Chinese psyche for centuries prior to this.

The earliest recorded reference to Yin Yang is in the *I Ching*, the Book of Changes. Traditionally the original trigrams described in the *I Ching* are said to have been discovered by Fu Hsi (the Chinese equivalent of Adam) drawn on the back of a tortoise which crawled out of the Yellow River. Legend puts this date at around 5000 BC. Dates of commentaries are rather more certain; those of King Wen and his son the Duke of Chu being around 1144 BC, and one by Confucius (551–479 BC). The high point in *I Ching* studies was reached during the Han Dynasty, at which time the separate theories of medicine from the North and South of China were being joined together to form a comprehensive whole.

Five Element theory (often translated as Five Phases or Five Transformations) was developed later than Yin Yang, initially as an independent theory. It had wide influence in the arts, culture and politics. Five Element theory was merged with Yin Yang theory by Tsou Yen (c. 340–260 BC) leader of the Yin Yang philosophical school. Further classic texts such as *The Spiritual Axis*, *The Classic of Difficulties*, and *The Pulse Classic* ensued, bringing together the accumulated knowledge, research, philosophical development and practical experience of medical practitioners over the centuries. These, together with other works, form a very large body of literature on oriental medical theory and practice which are still read, respected and referred to as authority even in the twentieth century.

18

ORIENTAL MEDICAL THEORY
SPREADS TO JAPAN

The migration of these ideas to Japan did not commence until about the sixth century AD. Buddhism was introduced to Japan somewhere between AD 538 and 552, and with it came an influx of Chinese philosophy and culture. Taoism, Buddhism and Confucianism were the three main strands in Chinese thought, each combining and weaving together in different measure the concepts of Tao and Yin Yang. Trading and diplomatic missions increased the contact between Japan and China and in AD 608 Prince Shotuku sent a delegation of Japanese students to China to learn Chinese culture and medicine. By AD 984 the oldest existing Japanese medical text had been written: the 30 volume *Ishinho* by Tamba Yasuyori.

However, the great flowering of oriental medicine took place during the Edo Period (1603–1868) as the Tokugawa Shoguns turned their backs on the European influence of the Dutch and Portuguese and fostered the development of oriental traditions. They decreed that massage was a profession which could be taken up by the blind, since their sense of touch is extra sensitive. Inevitably, since educational opportunities for the blind were restricted, the medical aspects' of Anma began to be lost. Masseurs became less qualified than doctors and were therefore less highly regarded. Also, doctors were using the whole range of medical techniques with an emphasis on herbal treatment which, because of the ingestion of substances into the body, required rigorous training. Doctors and herbalists were seen as working more in the realm of medicine, while Anma became associated principally with relaxation and pleasure.

It is interesting to note, however, that the medical application of massage technique was retained in the area of pregnancy and childbirth, by the use of a very specifically Japanese form of abdominal treatment known as *Ampuku*. Ampuku is a specialized form of abdominal massage which has been used medicinally for centuries. It is effective in the treatment of many conditions but has particular application to gynaecological problems and childbirth. This practice is noted in the chapter on 'Midwifery in Japan' in *The Women* by Ploss & Bartels. A Doctor Sigen Kangawa wrote a book on obstetrics called the *San-ron*, the 'Description of Birth' in 1765. Kangawa

> made use of *ampuku* for obstetrics, a massage in use in Japan from ancient times which is said to help various maladies. He introduced it as a methodical, careful and gentle pressure or palpation of the abdomen for the diagnosis of pregnancy, as well as for the acceleration of delivery and for the elimination of various ills of pregnant women.

THE MODERN HISTORY OF SHIATSU

The devaluation of Anma massage as a form of medical treatment continued into the early twentieth century when there was a revival signalling the start of the modern history of Shiatsu. The catalyst for this revival was the publication in 1919 of a book entitled *Shiatsu Ho* by Tamai Tempaku. He practised Anma, Ampuku and Do-in, and in addition had made considerable studies in Western anatomy, physiology and massage. His book brought together these various strands and reintegrated the spiritual dimension of healing into body-work. It seems that his work was influential in stimulating further research, and many of those instrumental in the development of Shiatsu studied under him, notably Katsusuke Serizawa, Tokujiro Namikoshi and Shizuto Masunaga. To those of us looking back from the perspective of the late twentieth century and from a Western point of view, it seems that these three men, Namikoshi, Masunaga and Serizawa, were the most influential figures in the development and current popularity of Shiatsu.

Namikoshi-style Shiatsu

Namikoshi used rubbing and pressing techniques to help his mother who was afflicted with arthritis. He trained in Anma but continued to develop his own method and in 1925 opened the Shiatsu Institute of Therapy in Hokkaido. By 1940 he had transferred his centre to Tokyo where he established the Japan Shiatsu Institute. In 1955 Shiatsu was legally approved as part of Anma massage and the Japan Shiatsu School was licensed by the Minister of Health and Welfare two years later. Shiatsu was finally recognized as a therapy in its own right as distinct from Anma and western (Swedish) massage in 1964. Quite when the term *Shiatsu* was actually coined is not recorded in any written text, but it is undoubtedly a modern word to distinguish the form from Anma and Ampuku.

Namikoshi's major contribution was the gaining of official recognition for Shiatsu, the establishment of a training school and his extensive teaching which spread information about Shiatsu throughout Japan and to the USA. It is perhaps ironic that in his eagerness to have Shiatsu accepted by the western scientific mind, Namikoshi removed all mention of meridians, energy and traditional theory from his work, and thus his style of practice tends to appeal less to the modern generation of bodywork students who are actively seeking a subtle, one might say spiritual, aspect to bring into their work.

Tokujiro Namikoshi's approach has been continued by his son Toru Namikoshi who spent seven years teaching Shiatsu in the USA and Europe, and set down a comprehensive guide to this style in his book *The Complete Book of Shiatsu Therapy*. The techniques used in this form of Shiatsu are very physical and symptomatic, working largely on neuro-muscular points and around areas of pain.

The theoretical basis of Namikoshi-style Shiatsu depends upon detailed knowledge of the muscular, skeletal, nervous and endocrine systems, in short a very western approach, while the overall view on good health is somewhat more traditional and includes advice on good diet, elimination, exercise and laughter.

Zen Shiatsu

The second figure to influence Shiatsu in the later part of the twentieth century was Shizuto Masunaga. Where Namikoshi uses pressure technique and places no reliance on the meridian system, Masunaga brought Shiatsu firmly back into the realms of traditional oriental theory. Being a psychologist by training, Masunaga was very interested in the psychological, emotional and spiritual aspects of energy imbalance. He pioneered a system, usually referred to as Zen Shiatsu, which seeks to discover which of the 'life aspects' described by the meridian functions is disturbed, and uses a specific theory of energy balance (known as kyo-jitsu theory) to interpret this. Masunaga extended the traditional acupuncture meridians to form a more complex network of traditional and 'supplementary' meridians which give the practitioner increased scope to work creatively with the body's energy. He also developed a detailed and specific form of abdominal diagnosis. Since Masunaga's death his work has been continued and developed by several teachers in Japan and in the West, and Zen Shiatsu is now widely practised in the USA and Britain, where research using Masunaga's methods and models is extending our understanding of energy manifestation and how to manipulate Ki.

Tsubo Therapy

Katsusuke Serizawa concentrated his research into the nature and effects of the tsubo, that is, the points themselves. Using the traditional concepts of oriental medicine he studied the location and functions of the tsubo found on the meridians, and utilizing modern electrical methods of measurement he tested the meridians and their tsubo to prove their existence scientifically. In recognition of this important experimental research he was awarded a Doctor of Medicine degree in 1961. Tsubo Therapy, as Serizawa calls his method of treatment, concentrates very much on the therapeutic qualities of the points, and can use massage, pressure, acupuncture, moxa or any of the more modern stimulating gadgets that are currently on the market. This is a little different in approach from standard Shiatsu, but a derivation of this style, Acupressure Shiatsu, is practised in the USA utilizing various acupuncture classifications of points.

OTHER DIFFERENT FORMS AND STYLES OF SHIATSU

So we can see that Shiatsu, like many other disciplines, has its own particular history which has led different individuals to focus upon different aspects of the overall therapy. Several distinctive styles have been given specific names denoting their theoretical approach or their originator. We have already mentioned Namikoshi style, Zen Shiatsu, and Acupressure Shiatsu or Tsubo Therapy. In addition to these, the other forms generally acknowledged are Macrobiotic Shiatsu, which incorporates Barefoot Shiatsu and integrates the use of traditional meridians with the dietary and lifestyle theories of George Ohsawa, Michio Kushi and Shizuko Yamamoto. Ohashiatsu is the method used by Wataru Ohashi, incorporating aspects of Zen Shiatsu and Namikoshi style with the use of traditional meridians. Five Element Shiatsu is similar in theory and methodology to Five Element Acupuncture, using the dynamic of the Five Elements and a classification of points according to their element influence: this form is mostly practised in the USA. Nippon Shiatsu is again an American designation basically comprising Namikoshi's method with knowledge of the traditional meridians. As well as these distinctive styles, some Shiatsu practitioners have been greatly influenced by Traditional Chinese Medicine (TCM), a specific theory of acupuncture and herbalism. They tend to use TCM as a theoretical model although their actual technique is usually closer to Zen or Namikoshi Shiatsu than to modern Chinese massage, Tui-Na.

COMMON STRANDS WITHIN SHIATSU

From the previous paragraphs we may have the impression that Shiatsu is very much divided, but in fact there is a common core of technique running through all approaches which is summed up in the therapy's name, 'Shiatsu', which means 'finger pressure'. Shiatsu is about pressure on the body; whether the practitioner describes his theoretical basis in terms of meridians and tsubo or trigger/neuro-muscular points, the fact remains that Shiatsu involves pressing, rubbing and stretching the body in order to revitalize it. For this reason we find that generally practitioners and students can use more than one approach quite compatibly within their treatment. Indeed in Britain the regulatory organization for Shiatsu, the Shiatsu Society, actively encourages cross-fertilization of ideas and therapeutic approaches by requiring practitioners who wish to go onto its professional register to have studied more than one style of Shiatsu. This is to give students an understanding of other ways of working, and thus to avoid the rifts which have from time to time dogged the progress of other therapies.

In Japan, Shiatsu remains popular with the older generation who have retained the more traditional ways, while younger people seem to prefer Western medicine. However, forms of Shiatsu are widely taught by the martial arts schools as the healing aspect of their disciplines. In contrast, Shiatsu is growing in popularity in Britain, the USA, parts of Europe and Australasia where people are looking for a holistic way of bodywork which can incorporate a strong spiritual or esoteric element.

Shiatsu is a growing and developing discipline. Far from being trapped in the past or fossilized into set techniques, it is continuing to progress and push back the boundaries of our understanding of Ki energy and our ability to direct Ki for healing in the body. While acknowledging and respecting our ancient historical roots and the great teachers of the past, we can move forward using all kinds of methodology from the esoteric to the scientific to continue the development of Shiatsu as a living, dynamic therapy.

3

How Does Shiatsu Work?

The Tao begets the One,
the One begets the Two,
the Two beget the Three and
the Three beget the Ten thousand things.
All things are backed by the shade,
faced by the light
and harmonised by the immaterial breath.
                    Lao Tzu: *The Tao Te Ching*

KI

FROM VERY ANCIENT times the Chinese have considered the universe to be comprised of energy in various stages of vibration and manifestation. Modern quantum physicists are proving now in their laboratories what the ancient orientals have known for centuries, that Ki energy is found in the tiniest particles that make up the form and substance of our universe. Indeed those particles, the building blocks of all matter and form, are themselves no more than Ki in vibration. Ki refers to energy in the very widest sense; it is everywhere, in everything, never ending or beginning, it encompasses time, space, matter, form, movement. Everything is Ki and Ki is everything. Everything that we can conceive of is merely Ki manifesting in a different form, ranging from the most subtle levels; spirit, thought, aura, love, light, air, to the denser and material substances: earth, rock, metal, animate beings.

For those of us brought up in western culture this concept of the whole universe being made essentially of the same 'stuff' is an alien and difficult idea. However, if we look at some simple examples we can easily see how Ki as existence is constantly changing yet never ceasing to be. A drop of dew that condenses in the cool of night warms up and vaporizes during the day, rising to form a cloud, where it may freeze into a hailstone, fall to earth and melt back into water . . . A piece of wood is thrown on a fire, it burns and floats into the air as smoke and ash; the ash settles on the earth where it forms part of the soil and feeds a seed which becomes a tree, which is cut for firewood . . . These are two very simple examples of how things change in form and substance, yet the energy which constitutes them continues to exist.

A more complex and long-term illustration might be the creation of a human being through the sexual activity of a man and woman. The cluster of cells grows to form a perfect human body, which emerges into the world as a child. Within the maturing person cells are constantly dying and being renewed so that the full-grown adult is not the same substance in terms of flesh, blood and bone as the little child, yet they are the same person. Eventually they die and the body decomposes into the ground while the spirit returns to what the Chinese would term 'the Great Void'. (Shiatsu, by the way, does not have any views about the hereafter and is perfectly compatible with any religion or philosophical outlook.)

We can see from these examples that things in existence are in a continual state of transformation; even the processes of life, growth and death are themselves only changes of form at a very elementary cellular level. What is common to all is Ki. Ki is the energetic substance of all things, it is also the force underlying all change and movement. In short, our entire universe is composed of Ki manifesting in an infinite number of forms and stages of materialization. Ki is 'the One' referred to in the quotation by Lao Tzu at the start of this chapter, and it is interesting that most religions have an emphasis on the number one: the acknowledgement of one God, or the attaining of oneness.

26

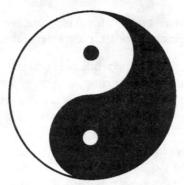

Fig. 1. Yin Yang symbol

YIN AND YANG

'The One begets the Two.' The Ki of the universe at the beginning of time differentiated into two forces, Yin and Yang. The quality of Yang was more rarified, immaterial and more vast, it therefore floated upwards to form the Heavens. Yin was more condensed and material, it sank down and created Earth. Thus the ancient Chinese philosophers explained the creation of the world.

The theory of Yin Yang describes how Ki differentiates into different qualities, and how these forces interact. As a theory Yin Yang dates from pre-Taoist times and is a view of the universe based upon centuries of experience and observation by the Chinese people. We should note that this is a *theory*, a human intellectual construction which we can use to describe and make sense of the real world as we experience it. Yin Yang is both a way of summing up the movement of Ki, describing how the universe works, and it is also a way of thinking. It is an all-encompassing theory and at the same time a simple tool which, once learnt, can be used to explain any number of phenomema, for example: why some people get on well together and others don't, why certain people tend towards a certain hobby or activity, how to choose the best food for you as an individual, why you may keep getting the same kind of health problem, how political and economic changes come about, how the moon affects the sea tides . . . and so on, the possibilities are endless.

If we look at the symbol for Yin Yang we can see that it illustrates the principles which are essential to the theory.

1. The circle symbolizes the wholeness and infinity of Ki, having neither beginning nor ending, and pervading everything.
2. The line dividing the two forces is a curved one, denoting movement and the constant flow of Yin into Yang and vice versa.
3. Within each colour is a dot of the opposing one. This shows that there are no absolutes and that everything contains the seeds of its opposite within it. Yin and Yang may be opposites, but they cannot exist without each other: there is no up without down, no hot without cold. Also each Yin and Yang can be further broken down relative to each other, therefore within hot we have tepid (more yin), and fiery hot (more yang), within cold moderately cold (more yang) and icy (more yin).
4. The two colours are in equal proportion, making a dynamic balance. When there is more of one aspect, there is less of the other, and at their extremes they transform into each other.

The dynamic of Yin Yang is therefore a very flexible and all embracing theory. Its qualities are not exclusive, but complementary and relative. Life is not black and white, but a scale of colours going from one end of the spectrum to the other and always changing.

The original meaning for Yin and Yang were 'the shady side of a hill' and 'the sunny side of a hill' respectively. Yin therefore was associated with darkness, coldness, resting, quietness. Yang was the opposite: light, heat, activity, movement. By the further association of Yang with Heaven and Yin with the Earth a whole series of qualities were assigned to each category, always bearing in mind that these are relative. The principal qualities are:

Yang	*Yin*
Heaven	Earth
light	dark
hot	cold
dry	damp

Sun	Moon
fire	water
active	passive
movement	rest
hard	soft
expansion	contraction
rising	sinking
immaterial	material
male	female

In regard to medicine, Yin Yang is the fundamental principle used to diagnose the individual's state of Ki and to describe the nature and location of illness.

Within the *body* Yin and Yang qualities can be categorized as follows:

Yang	*Yin*
back	front
outside of limbs	inside of limbs
surface	deep
exterior	interior
upper body	lower body
extrovert	introvert
more physical	more intellectual
left side	right side
acute	chronic

Yin Yang tends to be used as an overall general guide to the state of a person's Ki. We all have a constitutional tendency to be either more Yin or more Yang in nature. If in the shorter term, however, either the Yin or the Yang forces greatly predominate in the body or mind, then there will be an imbalance, leading to symptoms of one sort or another. Using the above tables to give us a feel for the qualities of Yin and Yang we can see that Yang symptoms or imbalances generally speaking would include things like stress, tension, overactivity, fevers, 'blocked energy'. Yin patterns would involve tiredness, lethargy, feeling 'spaced out', chilliness, 'deficient energy'. Using Yin Yang theory we can sum up a person's constitution or long term tendencies, and their condition, or short term symptoms.

THE FIVE ELEMENTS

The Five Elements represent a further classification of Yin and Yang into different forms of Ki described by the qualities of Metal, Water, Wood, Fire and Earth. We should note that the word 'element' in English has a somewhat fixed connotation that is not present in the Chinese, hence the theory is often known by the alternative translations *Five Transformations* or *Five Phases*. The Elements themselves are in fact descriptions of Ki in different stages and processes of change. For practitioners of Shiatsu and other forms of oriental medicine, Five Elements is a very useful model to work with as it is more tangible and therefore easier to grasp than the sometimes nebulous feeling qualities of Yin Yang. Like Yin Yang, the Five Element view of the universe arose from observing the cycles of nature and categorizing the interaction of phenomena.

Five Element theory comprises two aspects; firstly the grouping together of things or phenomena with a similar energy quality into *correspondences*, and secondly the flow of energy between the Elements in very defined sequences or *cycles*.

Each Element has its own characteristic properties and qualities which we can understand on an intuitive and commonsense level. Wood energy, for example, is the rising, expanding and growing feeling we are aware of in the Spring when nature starts to waken from winter and begins the great surge of activity that starts the year. Fire quality is the ultimate Yang of high summer when nature is at its peak of growth; the trees are in full leaf and flowers bloom. Earth is the element of centre and balance where the energy starts to transform into a downwards movement; it is associated with late or Indian summer and also with the last few days of each season when the Ki of the season starts to change into the next. Metal energy is consolidating and inward moving, like the sap in the trees contracting in the autumn. It condenses things into their constituent parts and creates the boundaries which define them; like an autumn mist lying in a valley, created by the condensation of water but unable to rise up and transform itself by evaporation. Water is the ultimate Yin; the quiet, cold, resting time of Winter. It has a waiting, still quality which could be described as 'stored potential', yet it is always capable of flexibility (think of water filling up any shape of vessel) and has great power (think of the devastation left by floods).

The Five Element *correspondences* group together phenomena which are seen to have a similar energy quality, rather like a group of musical instruments all playing the same note.

Table of general correspondences

Element	Wood	Fire	Earth	Metal	Water
season	Spring	Summer	Late Summer	Autumn	Winter
process	birth	growth	transformation	harvest	storage
climate	wind	heat	humidity	dryness	cold
colour	green	red	yellow	white	black/blue

When applied to the realm of the human body, mind and spirit Five Elements can be an invaluable tool in pinpointing where and how the body's Ki has become imbalanced.

Table of human correspondences

Element	Wood	Fire	Earth	Metal	Water
Yin organ	Liver	Heart/ Heart Governor	Spleen	Lungs	Kidney
Yang organ	Gall bladder	Small Intestine Triple Heater	Stomach	Large Intestine	Bladder
tissue	muscles	blood vessels	flesh	skin	bones
sense	sight	speech	taste	smell	hearing
taste	sour	bitter	sweet	spicy	salty
sound	shouting	laughing	singing	crying	groaning
positive emotion	humour	joy	sympathy	positivity	courage
negative emotion	anger	hysteria	self-pity	grief/ melancholy	fear/fright
capacity	planning	spiritual awareness	ideas/ opinions	elimination	ambition/ willpower

31

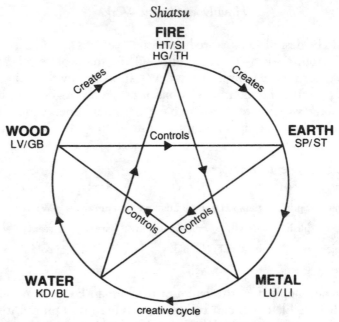

Fig. 2.   *Five Elements Shen & Ko cycles*

We shall look at the practical application of the Five Element correspondences a little further on in this chapter and in the next chapter when we look at some case histories.

The second important aspect of Five Element theory is its very specific description of energy flow, summed up in the Creative (Shen) and Control (Ko) cycles (Figure 2). On the Creative cycle, each element creates the next, so Wood creates Fire, which creates Earth and so on round the circle. The cycle of the seasons is a good example of this: in Spring (Wood energy time) the energy of the earth rises and bursts into the high activity of Summer (Fire), which then transforms to Indian summer (Earth time). Indian summer mellows to the harvest time of Autumn (Metal) and then the Ki of the earth rests and stores itself during the Winter (Water energy time) before beginning the whole process again in the Spring. The Control cycle is the five pointed star in Figure 2 and shows the way in which the elements also limit each other to restrain the otherwise infinite process of increasing. Again we can look to nature to explain the mechanisms at work here: Water puts out Fire, Fire melts Metal, Metal cuts Wood, Wood (trees) stabilizes the Earth, Earth dams up Water.

HOW KI WORKS IN THE BODY

When we apply the generalized theories of Yin Yang and the Five Elements to the body they provide us with a very apt description of the ways in which Ki flows and balances. Good health requires a free and harmonious flow of Ki throughout all parts of the body, rather like a network of rivers and streams flowing steadily through the countryside. And because the mind, emotions and spirit are merely a less dense aspect of the individual's material bodily Ki, when Ki is flowing smoothly in the body it is also balanced in mind and spirit. This is the essence of the holistic approach of oriental medicine and Shiatsu in particular; that we can feel the imbalance of Ki by touching the body, no matter at which level (physical, emotional, spiritual) the imbalance is occurring, and that by the use of technique – pressure, rubbing and stretching – we can realign the imbalanced Ki.

Ki comes to us from three basic sources. *Original Ki* comes from our parents; we could say it is our genetic inheritance and our basic constitution. *Grain Ki* is the Ki we ingest from our food. *Air Ki* is derived through breathing. These three together comprise our overall Ki quality.

Ki has five basic functions in the body:

1. *Movement*: in other words any form of activity whether physical or mental, voluntary or involuntary.
2. *Protection*: it protects the body from outside influences such as cold, wind, infections and so on.
3. *Warmth*: Ki keeps all parts of the body warm, regulating overall temperature and also peripheral circulation.
4. *Transformation*: it is Ki that changes food into the various building blocks which we need for good health.
5. *Retention*: keeping the organs in their proper places, preventing prolapse, holding blood in the blood vessels, and so on.

Chinese acupuncture theory has a whole complex classification of different manifestations of Ki in the body-mind, which practitioners of Shiatsu are aware of, but it is unnecessary for us to go into them here. The only two aspects of Ki which will be useful for us to note are *Jing* and *Shen*. These are Chinese terms and in Shiatsu we tend to use these rather than the Japanese equivalent. Jing is the essential energy which governs the long term processes of growth, maturation and death. It is responsible for our ability to have children and the pace at which we age. Jing resides in the Kidneys. Shen is translated as either the 'spirit' or the 'mind' but in reality encompasses both of these facets of ourselves. It is to do with our emotions and also the human awareness and consciousness which make up our individual personality. The Shen is said to reside in the Heart.

CAUSES OF IMBALANCE

What is it that causes Ki to become imbalanced or disturbed in the body-mind? In reality there is never one cause, but a network of factors which may combine to manifest in a particular pattern of imbalance. Oriental medicine basically classifies the sources of imbalance into internal or emotional factors, external or climactic factors, and lifestyle or miscellaneous factors.

The seven principal emotions are: *joy, sadness, fear, fright, worry, overthinking* and *anger*. Each is associated with a particular meridian, for example; joy affects the Heart, anger affects the Liver, fear affects the Kidneys, and so on. These associations are detailed in the section on meridian imbalance further on in this chapter (page 39).

The external factors can be likened to weather conditions and indeed at the changing of the seasons or when there has been a drastic change in the weather, symptoms of illness will often appear. These symptoms very often have the same characteristics as the weather conditions which caused them. Again they have specific Element associations. For example: *Cold* affects the Water element and causes symptoms of chilliness and shivering. *Wind* produces symptoms which move about the body, and is associated with Wood element. *Heat* results in high temperatures, sweating and thirst, which are detrimental to the Fire element. *Dampness* creates discharges, mucus and heavy feelings in the head and limbs; the Earth

34

element is most affected. *Dryness* afflicts the Metal element, and the accompanying symptoms include a dry cough, cracked skin and constipation.

The miscellaneous factors are fairly self explanatory: lifestyle and stress, diet, level of physical and sexual activity, injuries, bites and stings, inappropriate medical treatment, and misuse of drugs.

By understanding the ways in which Ki can be disturbed in the first place, we can gather clues as to how to deal with the resulting imbalance.

THE MERIDIANS

Ki moves throughout the whole body, but in certain defined pathways flows in a more concentrated manner. These pathways are known as the *meridians*. The meridians form a continuous circuit of lines which allow the flow of different aspects of Ki all over the body. Each meridian is named after a physical organ, for example Heart meridian, Lung meridian, Bladder meridian. However the meridian does not just relate to the physical organ, but encompasses a whole constellation of meanings based round a particular *function*. Indeed the easiest way to define a meridian is in terms of function. Rather than think of the meridian as a pathway attached to an organ, we should look on the meridian as a concentration of a particular functional energetic quality in the body. Where it reaches its most intense point, there it creates a physical organ to carry out that function. Knowledge of where the meridians run has been developed through centuries of observation and clinical experience, and nowadays can be measured scientifically with electronic instruments. Shiatsu practitioners learn to feel the meridians through increased sensitivity of touch.

There are twelve meridians which run on both sides of the body and two central channels; as in Figure 3. The meridians are classified in Yin and Yang pairs by Element and according to their function. If you imagine someone standing with their arms stretched up to the sky, the Yang meridians run from the 'Great Yang' of Heaven down the back and outsides of the body, whereas the Yin meridians run from the 'Great Yin', the Earth, up the front and insides of the limbs. Each Element has a particular energetic quality which governs a particular function. This is carried out by a pair of meridians which are in effect the Yin and the Yang aspects of the same function or Ki quality, rather like two sides of the same coin. The following table shows the functions of the meridians using Zen Shiatsu theory (which I use in my practice). You may find it useful to refer back to the Five Element human correspondences table to see some of the connections (page 31).

Element	Meridian	Aspect	Function
Metal	Lung	Yin	Intake of Ki (air) & vitality
	Large Intestine	Yang	Elimination
Earth	Stomach	Yang	Intake of nourishment
	Spleen/Pancreas	Yin	Digestion & Transformation
Fire (primary)	Heart	Yin	Emotional/Spiritual Centre
	Small Intestine	Yang	Assimilation
Water	Bladder	Yang	Purification
	Kidneys	Yin	Impetus
Fire (secondary)	Heart Governor	Yin	Circulation
	Triple Heater	Yang	Protection
Wood	Gall bladder	Yang	Decision making & Distribution
	Liver	Yin	Control & planning, Detoxification

You will notice that the order in which the meridians are listed here is different from the order of the Five Elements flow using the Creative cycle. This is because in *meridian theory* Ki runs from one meridian to the next in a continuous loop, so the Lung meridian ends close to where Large Intestine starts; where Large Intestine finishes Stomach begins, and so on. Each meridian is also associated with a particular time of day when its energy is strongest. This can be a handy tool in diagnosis to pinpoint someone's strengths and weaknesses. For instance a night owl like myself who is happy working till 3am has fairly strong Gall bladder and Liver energy, but I always have a slump mid-afternoon between 3pm and 5pm which is Bladder time and definitely not my strongest meridian. The *Chinese Clock*

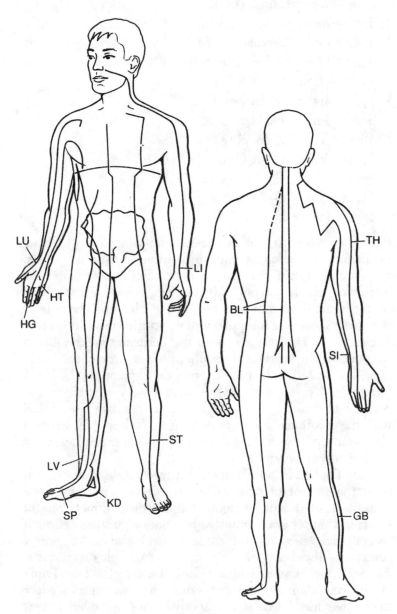

Fig. 3. The Meridians

cycle is the name for this aspect of theory and it runs as follows:

3am – 5am	Lungs (LU)
5am – 7am	Large Intestine (LI)
7am – 9am	Stomach (ST)
9am – 11am	Spleen/Pancreas (SP)
11am – 1pm	Heart (HT)
1pm – 3pm	Small Intestine (SI)
3pm – 5pm	Bladder (BL)
5pm – 7pm	Kidneys (KD)
7pm – 9pm	Heart Governor (HG)
9pm – 11pm	Triple Heater (TH)
11pm – 1am	Gall bladder (GB)
1am – 3am	Liver (LV)

Before we go on to look at the specific symptoms which we might find as a result of imbalance in any of the meridians, we should explain the nature and function of those two meridians which are not called after physical organs, that is the Heart Governor and the Triple Heater. The role of the Heart Governor is supplementary to the Heart. It is often known as the Heart Protector or the Pericardium (the sheath surrounding the heart) and its function is to protect the Heart as well as deal with the physical process of pumping the blood round the blood vessels. If we were to divide our western concept of 'heart' into two, the Heart meridian would deal with the emotional and compassionate, feeling side; whereas Heart Governor would regulate the physical organ heart and the circulatory system.

The Triple Heater (Triple Warmer/Triple Burner) has been the subject of much scholarly debate ever since the Chinese started writing about the medical dimensions of Ki. It is a rather unimaginative translation of 'three burning spaces' and refers to the three central *chakras* or energy centres in the body: the heart, the solar plexus and the *Tanden* (three fingers width below the navel). The Triple Heater has a much more generalized and widespread effect than other meridians. It is responsible for our overall temperature, rather like a thermostat, and it both produces and regulates heat throughout the body, as opposed to the Heart Governor which controls heat through the blood circulation. Although classified, with its pair Heart Governor, as Secondary Fire (Heart and Small Intestine being Primary Fire), the Triple Heater has a very close connection with the Water element, and is responsible for keeping all passageways in the body open thereby regulating the flow of liquids and Ki.

The *Yellow Emperor's Classic* likens the Upper Heater to a 'mist', the Middle Heater to a 'foam', and the Lower Heater to a 'swamp'. Largely each of the three Heaters is related to the organs found in each region, so the Upper Heater relates to Heart and Lungs, the Middle Heater to Stomach and Spleen and the Lower Heater to Liver, Kidneys, Bladder and Intestines. Zen Shiatsu takes these ideas from Chinese medicine and expands them in modern terms to say that Triple Heater also encompasses the functioning of the lymphatic system and the immune system.

Meridians and their related associations and imbalances

Let us now look at the detailed function of each meridian, its physical and psychological associations, and the sort of symptoms or conditions which would occur if it were out of balance. As I have said earlier, Shiatsu has several different theoretical approaches. The theory I am presenting here is the particular blend of Zen Shiatsu and Traditional Chinese Medicine which I use in my own practice. I find that in using theory I concentrate on the commonsense and practical applications rather than the esoteric or strictly classical. Therefore some of the categories below might, on the one hand, not be familiar to a Chinese acupuncturist, and on the other they might feel I have left out some functions. However, I find that Zen Shiatsu with its tendency to refine ancient oriental theory and explain it in more modern physiological terms makes a very satisfactory system to work with. Certainly it seems to make sense to my patients when I use it to explain their condition. Again you may find it useful to refer back to the Five Element human correspondences table (page 31).

Lung

Function: *vitality*, intake of Ki from the air; being able to take in new influences.

Physical associations: lungs; nose; skin.

Physical imbalances: any breathing or lung disorder including asthma, emphysema & coughing, tightness in the chest; nasal congestion & sinus trouble; any skin problems, eczema, spots, dry skin.

Psychological associations: making boundaries and structures; positivity; expression of grief; feeling of self worth; self as an individual.

Psychological imbalances: isolation and withdrawing; depression, melancholy; negativity, lack of self worth.

Large Intestine

Function: *vitality*; elimination & excretion.

Physical associations: bowels; skin; nose; sinuses.

Physical imbalances: any problem relating to the large intestine including constipation, diarrhoea, irritable bowel syndrome, diverticulitis; skin problems; excessive secretion of mucus & catarrh.

Psychological associations: being able to 'let go'; boundaries between self and the outside.

Psychological imbalances: inability to 'let go', too much 'holding on' (physically and mentally); isolation; rigidity or negativity in thinking and outlook.

Stomach

Function: *nurturing*; intake of food & other forms of nourishment (for example: emotional, social); beginning to break down food.

Physical associations: stomach and the upper digestive passages; flesh; chewing; mouth & lips; appetite mechanism; breasts and ovaries; any cyclical process such as menstrual, sleep, appetite cycles.

Physical imbalances: all stomach disorders including duodenal ulcer, hiatus hernia, indigestion, nausea & vomiting; weight problems; mouth ulcers; appetite disorders, overeating, anorexia nervosa; mastitis & breastfeeding problems; ovarian cysts, fibroids, endometriosis, prolapses; irregular bodily cycles.

Psychological associations: thinking, ideas & opinions; the mind and intellect; being 'grounded' and feeling in harmony with the earth; home and family; sympathy; mothering.
Psychological imbalances: too much thinking or studying, worrying, mental confusion, obsession & dogma; feeling ungrounded, instability, anxiety; not feeling at home anywhere; self-pity; fussing, not being nurtured.

Spleen/Pancreas

Function: *nurturing*; transportation and transformation of Ki; digestion; reproductive cycles.
Physical associations: secretion of digestive enzymes & the process of digestion; appetite; flesh and fat; menstrual cycle; controlling blood and keeping it in the blood vessels.
Physical imbalances: any digestive problems involving either insufficient or excessive secretion of digestive enzymes, including diabetes and hypoglycaemia; overeating or lack of appetite; weight problems; irregular, painful, or heavy periods, lack of periods; anaemia and bleeding disorders.
Psychological associations: as for Stomach.
Psychological imbalances: as for Stomach.

Heart

Function: *awareness*; our emotional centre through which we interpret our environment; blood circulation.
Physical associations: heart organ; central nervous system; tongue & speech; sweat.
Physical imbalances: heart disease and circulatory problems (note: this is usually more the province of the Heart Governor, but is also present in Heart); palpitations; speech disorders including stammering; excessive sweating (often at night).
Psychological associations: Heart houses the Shen which is the spirit and mind, that which characterizes us as human beings; human consciousness, awareness, compassion; emotions & emotional stability; joy, laughter; ability to express oneself, communication; sleep; long term memory.
Psychological imbalances: lack of compassion & empathy, personality disorders, mental restlessness; emotional instability, lack of emotion, inappropriate emotional response; hysteria; speech problems and inability to communicate; insomnia, dream-disturbed sleep; memory problems.

Small Intestine
Function: *assimilation*; absorption of nutrients into the blood; separation of that which is useful to the body-mind from that which is not (classically known as 'separating the pure from the impure').

Physical associations: small intestine, physical passage of nutrients from the digestive tract through the cell walls into the bloodstream.

Physical imbalances: poor absorption of nutrients, intestinal gas, abdominal pain, anaemia.

Psychological associations: clarity of judgement (separating one thing from another); dealing with mental anxiety, emotional excitement and shock; determination.

Psychological imbalances: inability to make decisions, cloudy judgement; inappropriate reaction to shock.

Bladder
Function: *purification*; storage and excretion of urine.

Physical associations: urinary system; water metabolism; bones & teeth; head hair; ears; the spinal column; autonomic nervous system.

Physical imbalances: any urinary problems including incontinence, urine retention, enlarged prostate; bone diseases including osteoporosis & some forms of arthritis; poor teeth; premature balding or grey hair; hearing problems & vertigo; lower back pain or weakness; overactivity of either sympathetic or parasympathetic division of the autonomic nervous system resulting in inappropriate reaction to stress, inability to relax, being too 'laid back'.

Psychological associations: fluidity; courage.

Psychological imbalances: restlessness; fearfulness & timidity, recklessness.

Kidneys
Function: *impetus*; will-power and progress in life; governs reproduction and sexual activity; houses the Jing.

Physical associations: the kidneys; the endocrine system, hormones, the reproductive system, sexual activity; overall potential and pace of lifespan; overall level of energy for activity; water metabolism; ears; bones & teeth; lower back; genetic inheritance.

Physical imbalances: any kidney disorders; hormonal and endocrine disturbances, all reproductive and sexual problems; irregularities in normal physical development such as growth, onset of puberty, premature ageing; chronic tiredness, exhaustion; fluid retention and water metabolism problems; hearing and balance problems, stumbling, being accident prone; weak bones & teeth; weakness, coldness or pain in the lower back; congenital & hereditary diseases.

Psychological associations: will-power, ability to go forward in life; ancestral Ki, genetic inheritance; courage; fluidity of emotions; short-term memory.

Psychological imbalances: lack of determination and ability to go forward in life; inherited psychological conditions; fear & phobias; restlessness & impatience; forgetfulness.

Heart Governor

Function: circulation; protects the heart; governs the blood circulation system.

Physical associations: the heart organ; arteries, veins; blood pressure.

Physical imbalances: heart disease; circulatory disorders including hardening of the arteries, varicose veins, poor circulation; blood pressure disorders; tightness in the chest, angina, palpitations.

Psychological associations: protection of the emotions & the Shen; social relations; sleep & dreams.

Psychological imbalances: overprotected or overprotective, emotionally vulnerable; nervous in social situations; insomnia, excessive or disturbed dreaming.

Triple Heater

Function: protection: harmonizes the generalized functions of the Upper, Middle, and Lower Heaters; the body's thermostat; protects the body's immunity via the lymphatic system; controls the opening of the waterways.

Physical associations: the Upper Heater is the Heart & Lungs regulating circulation and breathing, the Middle Heater is the Stomach & Spleen dealing with digestion and transportation, the Lower Heater consists of Kidneys, Bladder, Liver, Small & Large Intestines which are responsible for the separation of clean, useable fluid and food from the dirty parts which are then excreted; regulation of body temperature; lymphatic system, immune system.

Physical imbalances: lack of harmony between the three Heaters and their interrelated functions; poor heat regulation, poor circulation, overall chilliness or overheating; lymphatic problems, fluid & toxin retention; immune system disorders, allergies, lack of resistance to infections or illness.

Psychological associations: social interaction; emotional protection.

Psychological imbalances: lack of warmth socially; overprotective or overprotected.

Gall Bladder

Function: storage & distribution; stores & secretes bile; governs smooth movement of the body; controls judgement.

Physical associations: gall bladder; sides of the body; joints, muscles & tendons; digestion of fats; eyes.

Physical imbalances: gall stones & gall bladder problems; stiffness in movements, lack of physical flexibility, some forms of arthritis; lack of bile, biliousness, indigestion, poor digestion of fats; any eye problems, short & long sight; stiffness in neck and shoulders, migraine headaches; tiredness through overwork.

Psychological associations: decision making; creativity and initiative; hardworking, tenacious, responsible; good humour, anger, irritability.

Psychological imbalances: indecision; inability to turn plans into action, lack of creativity; tendency to work until exhausted, attention to detail, takes on too much responsibility; frustration, bitterness, impatient, constantly irritated.

Liver

Function: control: detoxification; storage; distribution; smooth body movement; harmonizes the emotions; planning.

Physical associations: liver; storing blood; detoxifying blood; energy & blood sugar metabolism; muscles, tendons, ligaments; eyes.

Physical imbalances: jaundice, cirrhosis of the liver; any liver organ problem; excessive or scanty menstrual flow; difficulty with detoxification, migraine, biliousness, gout; tiredness, stagnation of energy; muscular pains & stiffness, joints, tendon & ligament problems, arthritis; any eye problems.

Psychological associations: control; planning, being far sighted; harmonious emotions; good humour, anger; hardworking.

Psychological imbalances: over-control or feeling of being out of control, overwork; excessive planning, inflexibility in thoughts, not seeing clearly how to proceed; suppressed emotion, frustration, repression; shouting, temper tantrums; either lacks determination or never gives up.

In addition to the twelve bilateral meridians we have the two central channels, the *Governing Vessel* and *Conception Vessel*.

Governing Vessel

Function: influences all the Yang meridians in the body and can be used to strengthen the Yang forces.

Associations: the spine; the brain; Yang aspects of the Kidney meridian.

Imbalances: backache; nervous disorders, tremors, epilepsy; lack of vitality, sexual disorders; work on the Governing Vessel can have the effect of lifting the spirits and clearing the mind.

Conception Vessel

Function: influences all the Yin meridians; reproductive system.

Associations: the abdomen, chest, lungs, throat & face; fertility, childbirth, menopause.

Imbalances: any reproductive problems, fibroids, lumps, hernia, coldness, weakness, lack of will power.

In the above tables certain very common symptoms of imbalance, like headache, back pain and anxiety, have not been included. This is because such symptoms may occur in any of the meridians depending on cause and location. Therefore, we would classify, for example, right-sided severe headache as being most likely to be caused by a Gall bladder imbalance, and would treat it quite differently from a muzzy, 'not quite here' frontal headache which might originate in a Spleen or Stomach imbalance. The same can be said for back pain and anxiety: identifying the site of the disturbance would give a guideline as to which meridian is out of balance.

DIAGNOSIS

How does the practitioner decide which meridians to concentrate on during the session? If we were to use the meridian functions and associations purely in a symptomatic way we might be able to choose a meridian or set of meridians to work on, but they might not be the most appropriate ones for the patient, either in the long or the short term. What we use, therefore, is a framework of four methods of diagnosis in order to arrive at a conclusion about the patient's constitution (that is, his inherited and long-term tendencies), his condition (his short term state of health) and a description of the Ki imbalance found. This last is summed up using whichever theory of Ki movement or dynamics the practitioner finds most applicable in practice. The most common theories used in Shiatsu diagnosis to describe what the Ki is actually doing are: the Five Elements cycles, Kyo-jitsu theory (from Zen Shiatsu) and the Eight Principles (used widely by traditional Chinese acupuncturists).

Before we look at these in a little more detail, let us go back to the four forms of diagnosis mentioned earlier. These are:

1. *Asking questions*: which involves taking down a case history with details of their current state of health together with finding out about their general personality, likes and dislikes, and so on.
2. *Observation*: noting their general demeanour, posture, the colours they wear, lines, features and colours on the face. Observation would also include the intuitive feel picked up from them.
3. *Hearing and smelling*: this refers to listening to the tone of voice they use, whether sing-song, shouting, monotonous, weepy or groaning (these are Five Elements classifications). It also refers to the particular individual smell they give off, which has nothing to do with the aftershave or deodorant they are wearing. (I prefer my patients not to wear strongly perfumed products when they come for treatment as they

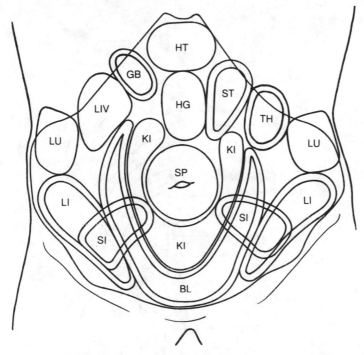

Fig. 4. Hara diagnosis map

mask the individual's own personal scent, and also tend to be unpleasantly overpowering for people who are sensitive to smell.)

4. *Touch*: this is the most important diagnostic tool in Shiatsu. There are certain well-defined areas where the practitioner can feel the quality of Ki in the meridians very clearly.

The most commonly used method of touch diagnosis in Shiatsu is *hara diagnosis*, although some practitioners would choose back diagnosis or pulses as their primary means of diagnosis. The hara has specific areas, rather like a map, which when palpated give feedback about the state of Ki in the meridian related to each area. We use the hara because it tends to be relatively protected and untouched and therefore gives a clear reading of the body's Ki status.

In the same way we have a map of the back with areas corresponding to meridians. There are also certain points on the front and back known as Bo points and Yu points

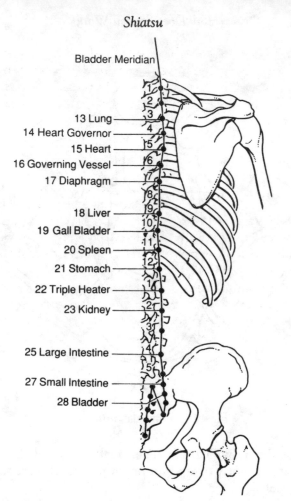

Bladder Meridian

13 Lung
14 Heart Governor
15 Heart
16 Governing Vessel
17 Diaphragm

18 Liver
19 Gall Bladder
20 Spleen
21 Stomach
22 Triple Heater
23 Kidney

25 Large Intestine

27 Small Intestine

28 Bladder

Fig. 5. The Yu Points (also known as Associated Effect Points or Back Transporting Points)

respectively, which when pressed may be tender or feel hard or soft; each of these points is associated with an individual meridian (Figure 5).

Another method of touch diagnosis is using the pulses found on the radial artery; again there is a position for each of the meridians and the quality of the pulse tells the practitioner what is happening with that particular meridian. Finally, there is the feel of the meridians themselves and how the Ki manifests in them.

The diagnosis reached by the four forms can be explained using whichever theory of Ki flow the practitioner finds most appropriate to work with. Most practitioners have a working knowledge of more than one system. Here are the major ones:

Five Element Cycles

This refers to the Creative and Control cycles described earlier in the chapter. If Ki is balanced throughout the body-mind it will flow smoothly round both cycles. If, however, it is disturbed anywhere then blockages and weaknesses will occur in patterns that follow the Creative and Control cycles.

Here is a simple example. If someone has strong ambition and will-power (Water) they will tend to push themselves and overtax the autonomic nervous system resulting in stress and inability to relax – this is an excessive Water condition. This excess is then pushed round the Creative cycle to the Wood element where it may manifest as headaches, irritability, overwork, tendency to drink too much alcohol and constant

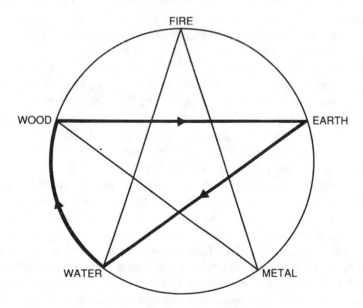

Fig. 6. A pattern of imbalance in water, Wood and Earth elements.

49

planning. Using the Control cycle, the excessive Wood would then typically restrain the Earth element too much, causing possible indigestion, stomach ulcers, and swings of high and low energy through the day – these are symptoms of low Earth energy. The Earth would have insufficient energy to control the Water and so the whole round would start again. Doesn't this sound like a typical overworked businessman? (See Figure 6.)

Of course this is a relative simplification since all the Elements would be involved as they are all related. Just as a stone dropped in a pool causes ripples over the whole surface, so any Ki disturbance results in repercussions throughout the whole body-mind.

Kyo-jitsu Theory

Masunaga's theory of kyo and jitsu illustrates the energetic distortion occurring in the body in terms of the dynamic interaction of Yin and Yang. Kyo is the more Yin quality; to the touch it feels either soft and empty, or stiff and resistant. Its overall characteristic is unresponsive. Jitsu on the other hand is more Yang in nature. It feels hard and full, bouncy and active. Its principal characteristic is responsive. Kyo and jitsu are always linked together in an energetic relationship in which the kyo causes the jitsu. The classic example of this is when we are hungry (empty and therefore kyo) we go off and find ourselves something to eat (activity, which is jitsu) and thus bring ourselves back to a comfortable balance. By working on the kyo, the cause or need, we can balance the jitsu. This system has a considerable amount of flexibility since any meridian could be in a causal energetic relationship with another. However, it is rare to find meridians within the same Element in a kyo-jitsu relationship as they have a similar Ki quality and therefore could not be both high and low in energy at the same time.

As an example of kyo-jitsu theory, let us imagine a person who has spent several years nursing a demanding elderly relative who has recently died. They have expended a great deal of caring, compassion and emotional energy in difficult circumstances, perhaps having to contend with the demands of their own growing family too, resulting in an emptiness (kyo) in the Heart meridian. On the death of their relative, our patient finds they feel stuck and unable to express their grief. Not only this, but they now feel unwilling to go out and meet people again after so much time at home, and to cap it all have developed constipation with occasional explosive diarrhoea – all symptoms of a jitsu Large Intestine. Therefore the energetic relationship here is Heart kyo, Large Intestine jitsu. The depletion of the emotional forces of the Heart resulting in an inability to express grief and in turn the inability to let go of their relative. Treatment would take the form of increasing the energy in the Heart, which would relax the Large Intestine and allow it to let go, solving both the emotional and physical problems.

You will notice that this is a more emotional and psychological example. This is because Zen Shiatsu tends to put an emphasis on the psycho-emotional causes of imbalance and acknowledges their close relationship with physical symptoms.

Eight Principles

This is another way of understanding and describing patterns of Ki imbalance and is used extensively in the Traditional Chinese Medicine (TCM) form of acupuncture. Some Shiatsu practitioners who are also acupuncturists make use of this theoretical model although the technique which follows on from it is possibly more applicable to acupuncture and the specific action of points than to Shiatsu. The Eight Principles are Yin/Yang, Interior/Exterior, Empty/Full, Cold/Hot. As we now know from the theory we have looked at so far, the six last categories are themselves subdivisions of Yin Yang. But again as we have noted previously, the *general* theory of Yin Yang as applied to all phenomena is sometimes difficult to use in the context of the complex human condition because of its very simplicity. Eight Principles therefore breaks Yin Yang down into more graspable parts to give a description of the energy *state*. It is interesting to note that in contrast to this, Five Element theory gives us more a description of energy *movement* or *process of change*.

Interior/Exterior describes the location of the imbalance. Empty/Full indicates whether Ki is deficient (similar to kyo), with chronic symptoms, weakness, tiredness, inactivity, and pain helped by pressure; or excessive (jitsu), with acute conditions involving restlessness, heavy breathing, and pain on pressure. Cold/Hot refers to the nature of the symptoms with Cold conditions resulting in feeling cold, pale face, no thirst, and Hot in overheating, fever, red face, thirst and constipation. Yin/Yang refers to the overall Yin Yang balance and to specific tendencies when imbalanced. For instance Yin tendencies would include being weak and tired, feeling cold, wanting to keep warm, lack of appetite, wanting to be held or touched. Yang signs include activity, restlessness, feeling hot, thirst, finding pressure or touch painful.

Each of these theoretical systems provides the Shiatsu practitioner with the means to be able to sum up where Ki may be distorted, and this in turn shows the means to treat the imbalance. It should be noted that these are all theories, in other words descriptions of reality – it is the practitioner's job to be able to use theory to fit reality, not to try to squeeze reality into a theory.

APPLICATION OF TECHNIQUE

Now that we have arrived at a diagnosis, a description of the Ki imbalance, what do we do about it? This is where we start to apply the techniques of Shiatsu. Because we are working with our hands on the body throughout the treatment we are going to be getting a lot of tactile feedback. I like to encourage my students to describe what they are feeling in creative or imaginative ways. This helps them to concentrate on the exact feel they are getting. In reading texts on Shiatsu and other forms of oriental medicine we tend to come across standard terms such as 'excessive' or 'deficient', which are useful as a starting point, but can limit our perception of touch if we stick rigidly with them.

In speaking of kyo we can say it is essentially unresponsive; in practice it may feel soft, like a jelly, a sinking feeling, nothing there to hold you out, or stiff, like a creaky board, with no give to it. Because the feeling in terms of *quantity* is 'not enough', we deal with kyo by putting more energy into the meridian in general and the tsubo that feel particularly empty; a process known as 'tonification'. This is effected by long, slow, holding pressure at medium to light depth, although always deep enough to contact the Ki. As a practitioner you can either hold passively and allow the receiver's Ki to focus into the point and fill it up, or you can consciously extend your own Ki into that tsubo using the hara and breathing techniques. The receiver will feel the sensation of your reaching and moving Ki in a kyo tsubo as a 'nice pain', a comforting pressure which feels supportive.

Jitsu is classically described as hard or responsive, but more creatively we may pick it up as bounding, bouncy, not letting you in, holding out, stuck or stagnant. In terms of quantity jitsu has too much Ki, so we want to encourage it to move on elsewhere by 'sedation'. Usually, in the ordinary way of speaking, to sedate someone would make us think of putting them to sleep, but in this case a better image is calming a hyperactive child to bring them back to a normal level of activity. Sedation techniques are fast, strong and deep, and may be painful if applied to a site of long term stagnation.

Being able to feel these different qualities is something which comes with practice. I feel that we all have the intuitive ability to know how to touch others appropriately, but it is an ability which can always be refined and developed. Two aids to sensitivity and intuition used in Shiatsu are the use of the hara and breathing.

The Hara

The abdomen, known as the hara, has great importance in Japanese culture and the eastern understanding of the Self. In the West we tend to think of ourselves in terms of our mind and our brain, with the body tacked on as an appendage. The oriental viewpoint puts the centre of ourself in the hara, with our vital energies, our seat of power and our intuitive faculties all based in this essential area. Although we talk about 'having a gut feeling' about something, or 'not having the guts' to do something, the Japanese concept of living and working from hara is very much wider than anything similar found in the West. Most of us are familiar with the feats of martial artists, breaking through multiple blocks of wood or throwing someone of weighty proportions to the ground. This is done by using the hara as a power centre and the effects can easily be seen. But the faculties of hara are also used in other Japanese arts: where to place a bloom in flower arranging or when to make the final brush stroke in a work of calligraphy. Using hara encompasses within it the idea of seeking perfection, or even enlightenment, through disciplined practice. There is no competitive element, for this is an inner, spiritual way. Developing the use of hara can be accomplished through many different media; meditation, exercise, martial arts, and of course Shiatsu. Using the power and sensitivity of hara gives Shiatsu practitioners the capacity to move beyond mere technique to powerful and compassionate healing in the largest sense of the word. Being based in hara increases our intuition and the sensitivity we have in our hands; it enables us to empathize with the receiver sufficiently to feel what they are feeling, yet gives us the distance not to be caught up in their problems and their symptoms.

Some simple exercises to help you get in touch with your own hara are included in Chapter 6.

Breathing

Use of the breath is another helpful tool in making Shiatsu more effective. The breath is in fact one of the most powerful tools at our disposal in life. If we breath deeply we energize ourselves and accept life to the full; if our breathing is shallow we lack vitality, almost a negation of being here at all. Inhalation fills us with new, clean Ki, energizing our entire system. Exhalation is the powerful and relaxing breath which allows us to relax and reach out to life. We all know that we sigh with relief, or to let go old feelings, but we may be less in touch with the powerful aspect of breathing out. Next time you are trying to undo a stuck jam jar, do it while breathing out and you will be surprised at the results! In Shiatsu we tend to apply pressure when we are breathing out and when the receiver is exhaling too. This allows us to visualize the flow of Ki through our hands more easily, and the receiver can relax and let go of any tension. By coordinating breathing in this way we can feel closer to each other and this empathy encourages the healing process.

THE POINTS THEMSELVES – TSUBO

The tsubo or classical acupuncture points are places where Ki accumulates on the meridians, rather like pools in a stream, and here it is easier to tap into Ki and manipulate it. The tsubo are numbered according to their position on the meridians, for example; KD1 – the first tsubo on the Kidney meridian. Modern scientific investigation has shown that the classical points are often situated at places where the body is weaker; at joints, in the depressions between muscles, where nerves run superficially. The electrical resistance of the skin is also lower at these points, pointing conclusively to the fact that 'something' is going on there, even if western medicine has not managed to define it yet. Energetically a tsubo is shaped like a vase with a narrow neck and wide belly. In order to contact the Ki in the point you must press in at ninety degrees. Each tsubo has specific properties or actions which may include reducing pain, moving Ki in specific directions, calming the mind, heating or cooling the body, or balancing the Elements. The theory of the action of points is obviously widely used in acupuncture, and although useful, in Shiatsu we tend to work more with the full meridian, feeling by intuition and sensitivity where the Ki disturbances are and working accordingly.

As well as the points on the meridians there are points which may become spontaneously painful; these are known as *Ahshi* or 'ouch!' points – and they usually do make people say 'ouch' when pressed! Medicine might define these as *trigger points* (of which more later). Within a Shiatsu session there is normally some work on Ahshi points around tender areas as well as work related to tsubo on the meridians. In Chapter 6 we shall look at some of the tsubo which can be used for first aid purposes using their therapeutic properties.

THE PHYSIOLOGY OF SHIATSU

So far we have looked at how Shiatsu works purely from an oriental point of view, but our western analytical and logical minds may still want the security of some sort of scientific explanation. Much of the scientific work which has been done on the effects of acupuncture, massage and meditation can be applied to the modus operandi of Shiatsu; and without going into great physiological detail, here are some of the basic explanations we can put forward for Shiatsu's undoubted effectiveness.

Research by Katsusuke Serizawa has established that the internal organs are linked to the skin, subcutaneous tissues and the muscles via the nervous system, and that by means of *nerve reflex actions* disturbances in the functioning of the internal organs can be felt on the surface of the body. His research has verified that the reverse is also true: that by stimulating a tsubo close to the spinal column corresponding to a particular spinal nerve, a reflex action is set up and the functioning of the organ fed by that nerve can be enhanced.

The nervous system is also involved in the explanation of the role of pressure in pain control. Pain is very often caused by chronic and inappropriate tension in the muscles. Without going into too much detail, let us say that there are nerve *reporting stations* which fire off messages to the central nervous system about the length of muscle fibres and the load being carried by them. Sometimes, due to habitual movements, poor posture or emotional tension, the reporting stations keep sending the message 'hold on' even when the reason for the original muscle action is no longer there. A very simple example is the woman who always carries a shoulder bag on one side. On looking at her we find that one shoulder is higher than the other because the muscles have got so accustomed to the constant tension needed to hold up the weight of the bag that she has forgotten to let go of it when the bag has been put down.

Pressure on tender points (known as *trigger points*) in her shoulder muscle will have two effects. Firstly opening up the capillaries, enhancing the flow of blood and lymph within the muscle so helping to remove toxins (such as lactic acid which causes cramp) which may have been contributing to the pain. Secondly, pressure inhibits the firing of messages from the *Golgi Tendon Organs* (which measure the tension or load being born by muscle fibres) to the *central nervous system* (CNS). This short circuiting of the messages means the CNS is no longer being told that it must continue to contract that muscle and relaxation results. All of this goes on, of course, outside our consciousness. Trigger points are points or areas of extreme sensitivity which on pressing produce referred pain in other locations. There has been considerable research into the theory and use of trigger points and these have been found to coincide very extensively with the locations of classical tsubo.

The secretion of *endorphins*, the body's natural painkillers, is also involved in the pain-relieving qualities of Shiatsu. Again there has been research in relation to acupuncture and endorphins, and pressure has been shown to be as effective if not more effective than needling.

Finally in looking at the overall calming and relaxing effect of Shiatsu we must acknowledge the role of the *autonomic nervous system* (ANS). The ANS is linked in to the action of smooth and cardiac muscle in the body, in other words dealing with the nervous functions which are not normally under our conscious control, such as the beating of the heart muscle, and the contraction of muscles needed to move food along the digestive tract. The two divisions of the ANS govern our response to our surroundings: the sympathetic division dealing with the 'flight or fight' reaction in which our body is geared up for stress while digestive and reproductive functions cease; the parasympathetic division reversing the effects of the sympathetic and inducing relaxation on a wide scale. The kind of supportive, comforting and pleasurable touch given in Shiatsu stimulates the parasympathetic division of the ANS, leading to a state of calmness and tranquillity.

We must not forget the importance of pleasant sensations when we talk of well-being. Sensory stimulation is vital to human well-being; babies can die from lack of physical contact; older people can feel cut off from the world, from themselves, and in consequence die away slowly for lack of human contact. It is interesting that there are more pathways sending touch sensation to the brain than those sending pain sensations. By creating pleasant tactile sensations away from the site of pain we may distract the brain from focusing on the pain and thus diminish its effects. Perhaps we could say the same on a wider scale: that by reaching out and touching someone in a caring and compassionate way we can lessen whatever pain is in their life and put a sense of well-being back in the forefront of their experience.

4

What Can Shiatsu Do For You?

HAVING EXPLAINED THE theories underlying Shiatsu, let us now look at the practical application of that theory in some real case histories. As I said in Chapter 1, Shiatsu can be used in the treatment of a wide range of conditions. Sometimes Shiatsu alone can balance up a person to the extent that their symptoms disappear. Sometimes it requires 'homework' in the form of exercises, changes of diet or habits, and looking at their attitudes along with Shiatsu to break the energetic patterns. Sometimes there are cases where Shiatsu is not effective, and then referral to another therapy is appropriate.

Like many other therapists, Shiatsu practitioners see themselves as educators, acting as catalysts to help patients help themselves. Your health is your responsibility and it is no good expecting your therapist, or your doctor, or anyone else to take that over. A good therapist of whatever kind will lead you to an understanding of your condition; what you then choose to do is up to you. The time that you spend in a Shiatsu treatment is about forty-five minutes to one hour – it is how you spend the rest of your time that determines your state of health. If I tell you that drinking ten cups of strong coffee per day is detrimental to your Kidney energy, and you continue to drink ten cups per day, no matter how much Shiatsu I apply, your Kidneys will still continue to be imbalanced! A holistic outlook with a good diet, activity balanced with relaxation, supportive social relationships and a sense of purpose in life is, of course, the ideal for all of us. We don't all achieve this.

If, however, we understand what we need, we can then go about seeking it out.

Practitioners find that patients come for treatment for one of two reasons: a) to deal with an existing health condition; b) to prevent future imbalance. Very often the second category arises from the first; in other words people come for treatment for a particular condition, find relief and then become aware of their part in preventing a further recurrence of the problem. Those people who have developed a sense of responsibility for their own health can be very inspiring for a therapist to work with since great changes and progress can be made.

As examples, I have chosen some of my own recent cases. They do not represent all the conditions Shiatsu can help with, but they give an idea of the kinds of imbalance for which Shiatsu is a very appropriate form of treatment. They also illustrate various aspects of the theory which we discussed in the previous chapter. For the sake of confidentiality, initials and some personal details have been changed.

STRESS AND TENSION HEADACHES

Mrs E started coming for Shiatsu two months before Christmas, her busiest time of year since she runs a toyshop. She described her problems as mainly stress from work which showed up as tension headaches and pain in the left shoulder. She was also going through the menopause with attendant symptoms, and suffered from depression at times having had a nervous breakdown several years ago. My main aim in treatment on a physical level was to work on her neck and shoulders to relieve the headaches, and on a psycho-emotional level to help her cope emotionally.

In terms of overall Yin Yang balance she had a tendency to swing between frantic activity (yang) and days of complete depression when she stayed in bed and did nothing (yin). In physical terms she was constitutionally quite yang with a strong square frame and heavy bones. However her current condition was fairly yin, with insufficient movement of Ki to ensure proper functioning of the internal organs, resulting in blockages of Ki in the upper body. (The upper body is more yang – refer back to the table of general body attributes of Yin Yang on page 29 – and therefore attracts yang Ki.) The impression on looking at her was rather top heavy: more yang and rigid at the shoulders and chest, yin and weak in the abdomen and legs. This last showed up in her feeling of being unable to exercise due to lack of energy in her legs. There was also weakness in the reproductive and lower digestive organs.

The predominant Five Element factors were Fire, Earth and Metal. Fire (Heart/Small Intestine: Heart Governor/Triple Heater) showed up in Mrs E's fluctuating emotional state, also hot flushes, night sweats and insomnia. Insomnia is attributed to a disturbance of the Shen and associated with the Heart. She also had a slight Heart defect, but I felt the emotional aspect of Fire was the important one in this case with the Heart energy needing special attention. Heart encapsulates our emotional life and our interaction with the world around us through our emotional responses. Mrs E would often arrive for treatment very agitated and 'high', and go away quite calm and peaceful – this was partly due to the relaxing effect of the treatment, but is also an indication of one of the attributes of imbalanced Fire; that it blazes up and then dies down in response to its environment. One of the primary aims in treatment was therefore to stabilize her Fire element so that she could react more appropriately to the undoubted stressful situations she found in her workplace, not blazing up or getting demoralized.

Earth (Stomach/Spleen) manifested in her being overweight, suffering from indigestion and belching, with cravings to eat chocolate (sweet taste) and junky carbohydrate comfort-type fast foods even though she knew these were not good for her. She also expressed a feeling of 'not having her feet on the ground', which is very typical of a weakness in Earth energy combined with unstable Fire: Fire not feeding steady energy round to Earth on the Creative cycle. We talked a lot about the nourishing function of Earth and the kinds of food that would be more nourishing to her. We settled on a regime of simple, quickly prepared meals since one of her reasons for eating junk food was having neither the time nor the inclination to cook during this short period of extraordinary work stress.

I felt that a lot of Mrs E's digestive problems were due to not chewing properly (again the time factor!), so I recommended ten chews per mouthful to activate the enzymes responsible for the breakdown of carbohydrate. She had read somewhere that she should chew each mouthful fifty times but had rejected that as totally impossible. I thought that by giving her an attainable number she would feel good about achieving it, and would in all probability chew a bit longer since she would at least be thinking about it. Her irregular periods, part of the natural process of going through the menopause, also come under the Earth category since Earth is responsible for fertility and time cycles in the body. But I did not feel this was an imbalance, just a description of what was going on with her as a natural part of ageing and therefore not a major factor in treatment.

Metallic associations (Lung/Large Intestine) in Mrs E's case were bloated intestines and constipation, excessive mucus production resulting in catarrh and congested sinuses, plus a depressive and somewhat negative melancholic outlook. Several times during her course of treatment she spoke of her 'inability to let go' both physically (constipation and inability to relax) and emotionally (holding on to old thoughts, feelings, even conversations). These are definite attributes of a jitsu Large Intestine where the body-mind is not able to eliminate.

Mrs E came for treatment weekly as she felt it 'kept her going' during this time of stress. She kept telling me she would be all right and quite different after Christmas. In the earlier sessions a pattern of Spleen kyo (the yin aspect of Earth being deficient) with Gall bladder jitsu (the yang aspect of Wood excessive) emerged. This I put down to largely psychological causes, since she was doing a great deal of planning and ordering of stock at work, with constant decision-making required (Wood), all of which had overworked and depleted the intellectual thinking aspects of Earth. This is an example of Wood controlling Earth.

Since I felt she was very much 'up in her head' besides experiencing a good deal of neck tension, shoulder pain and headaches, I spent a lot of time in the early sessions working on her Gall bladder meridian in the neck and shoulders with fairly strong pressure and muscle stretches on the trapezius muscle. This was balanced by slower holding on points on the Spleen meridian in the legs, especially below the ankle to try to 'get her feet on the ground'. After the second session I showed her how to do hara breathing, a simple exercise to centre one's energy in stressful and emotional situations. Later sessions threw up a consistent Heart kyo, Large Intestine jitsu pattern, which again seemed to be a description more of the state of her emotional Ki rather than her physical Ki. Heart was depleted due to the constant ups and downs of her reaction to stress at work and always being busy. Large Intestine jitsu represented her inability to let go of old emotional patterns along with the feeling that she *had* to react this way to all the stress at this time of year – she was also fairly constipated despite advice on diet which she accepted but may not always have followed.

In this phase the treatment sessions usually followed a pattern of holding palm pressure on the chest to stabilize and energize Heart Ki, and working on Heart and Large Instestine in both arm and leg (Masunaga's system of supplementary meridians has a branch of both Heart and Large Intestine in the leg). Again time was spent relaxing and releasing the shoulders as there were active trigger points in the trapezius and sternocleidomastoid muscles which were instrumental in her tension headaches. The trigger points coincided with tsubo on the Large Intestine meridian. The Yu points on the back for the Heart, Heart Governor and Triple Heater were often sore and I worked generally on loosening the back on all treatments.

Over the course of the treatment she made good progress and showed a real commitment to keeping herself as balanced as possible under the circumstances. The head and shoulder pain were decreased and if she came with a tension headache she usually left without it. Despite the fact that Large Intestine remained fairly stuck, her Heart energy improved and she commented that she felt more able to cope and was happier for longer periods, rather than swinging between being happy and miserable. We both saw her treatment as a 'holding operation' to get her through a difficult period in her working year, and I was pleased with her attitude of responsibility in wanting to do things to help herself rather than have me do all the work.

SHOULDER PAIN

Mr J was an entirely different case in that the problem and treatment were on a completely physical, symptomatic basis. He came with severe pain in his left shoulder which he had been suffering for several months. His doctor had had an x-ray taken which showed thinning of the bone and some arthritis at the end of the clavicle and scapula where the deltoid muscle originates. Mr J described the pain as like toothache, a bony pain not a muscular one, and more or less constant although worse after heavy lifting. The doctor had prescribed painkillers and also calcium for the bone deterioration, otherwise no other treatment. Going through Mr J's case history questionnaire produced very few symptoms or associations. Overall he was somewhat yin in quality; a quiet, not very active man of fine-boned slim build. He was generally in good health with a sensible diet and positive if unambitious outlook on life – altogether quite well balanced apart from the shoulder pain. Nothing outstanding appeared in the way of theoretical connections although his hara diagnosis often showed Kidney kyo, which would describe the lack of ambition in his work life. His home life seemed settled and content.

In treatment I concentrated on the shoulders which were tight on both sides on top of the trapezius muscle, and on the neck. I also worked on the supplementary Kidney meridian in the arm as well as traditional Kidney in the leg. This was to balance his general Ki and to draw energy away from the shoulders by working on the feet. The main part of each treatment was spent working directly on the site of pain as I found immediately that there was excessive muscle tone in the fibres of the deltoid muscle. Friction rubbing across the muscle and pressing the tsubo LI15 and TH14 (in the hollows formed at the top of the deltoid) was effective but rather sore. I felt the whole area needed to be released as Ki was very blocked there. On questioning Mr J, I discovered that part of his work involved carrying a heavy item, which he invariably did with the left arm bent and held away from the body, in other words using his deltoid muscle. What had occurred therefore was chronic tension in those muscle fibres which were unable to relax again when he was no longer using them. In order to short circuit the nervous impulses telling the muscle to keep contracting I used pressure and rubbing as described above. I also wanted to increase circulation into this local area so I applied indirect moxa (see Chapter 6) on LI15 and TH14 to heat up the area, energize blocked Ki and mobilize the shoulder joint. A week after the first treatment Mr J reported that there had only been one day when his shoulder had been painful. After four sessions the condition had gone except for the occasional twinge so he felt there was no need for further treatment although he will get in touch if it flares up again. We talked about the cause of the problem and he is varying his work habits so as to avoid the posture which created the problem in the first instance. A simple case of a localized physical problem with a simple physical solution.

PREMENSTRUAL SYNDROME AND LOWER BACK PAIN

Not all cases are so simple. When Mrs H first came to see me it was to help with her severe premenstrual symptoms and migraine. Over the months these came under control but she developed acute lower back pain on two occasions and has some problems with her marriage related to setting up her own business.

The initial symptoms were a short menstrual cycle with dark brown blood but no pain – indications of a kyo condition in the Spleen and Kidneys. From her point of view it was not so much the period that was the problem, but the week or so leading up to it during which she regularly suffered from acute depression and a feeling that she just wanted to give up and leave her husband, family and business. Coupled with that were ferocious one-sided headaches and digestive upset – two of the classic signs of migraine.

In the first treatments we concentrated on the Spleen and Liver meridians. Spleen because it governs the menstrual cycle and has some very effective points for alleviating menstrual problems (notably SP6, SP9 & SP10 – see page 82 for exact locations of these points). Also because she had spoken of her craving for sweet-tasting food before her period, an extremely common occurrence with a lot of women since the sweet taste goes along with the Earth element. A stuck or jitsu condition in the Liver is often the cause of migraine symptoms so we worked on the lower part of the Liver meridian, especially LV3, to bring her energy down out of her head. Liver also involves digestive disturbance, so we had a careful look at her diet and found that as well as sweet food she used to like oily foods.

On questioning her further I found that she sometimes went for several hours without food or drink, and then would feel that she just had to have a cup of tea with lots of sugar and some biscuits. Hypoglycaemia or low blood sugar is a condition where the body does not handle the balance of glucose in the blood very well, often leading to dizziness, irritability and headaches – both Spleen and Liver meridian are classically implicated in this disorder. By modifying Mrs H's dietary intake and its frequency we managed to decrease the incidence of migraine. Her treatment sessions were always carefully timed to coincide with the pre-menstrual time and this helped her to relax and also express some of the frustrations with her home situation which were contributing to her tight Liver.

Several months into her treatment Mrs H arrived one day with an acutely sore back. She had been practising some exercises and had gone too far, resulting in the deep back muscles going into spasm. Her posture was very protective and curled to one side, and she was afraid she had 'put her back out'. On careful examination I could assure her that all the bones were in place, but that the deep muscles on one side of the spinal column had seized up in response to the unaccustomed stretch. By applying palm pressure to the whole of the lumbar area and then gentle thumb pressure on the site of the pain the muscles began to relax. I used a particular technique to push up and down on the lateral processes of the spine (bony protrusions onto which the deep muscles attach) to ease out the muscles, and then with her lying on her back pressed her knees gently towards her chest. All of these measures proved effective, and she went away walking straight and feeling much less sore although not totally pain free. Subsequent treatments removed the pain altogether.

The energetic diagnosis of her back pain was Kidney kyo and Large Intestine jitsu – a combination of weakness and coldness in the upper lumbar area and tight holding at the lower lumbar and buttocks. The second episode of back pain several months later had the same pattern, but on this occasion Mrs H opened up and expressed a lot of anguish about feeling unsupported in her relationship and how she had suffered back pain during pregnancy when, again, she had felt unsupported. Working not just on the back but also the emotional centres enabled her to let go of many of the feelings she had been harbouring for years (a Large Intestine indication); she then felt strong enough to tackle her husband and communicate some of those feelings. Since that session her back has been better; as she said, it 'shifted a lot of stuff'. Treatment is ongoing, concentrating more on letting her get in touch with her fears (Kidney kyo) and being a listening ear. Feeling that she needed more specific advice on her relationship I encouraged her to go to a counsellor. As her Shiatsu practitioner I feel it is my role to support her through whatever decision she chooses to make and to help her Ki to remain balanced – other professionals are more qualified than I am to help her actually make that decision.

There are many other cases I could have chosen to illustrate how Shiatsu can help with the everyday ailments that can so disrupt our lives. The elderly lady with an arthritic hip who loves ballroom dancing and comes for pain relief; the dancer with irritable bowel syndrome; the gentleman whose asthma has improved to the extent that he can come off cortisone; the business executive with M.E.; the mother who takes care of everybody but herself . . . How much people get out of Shiatsu depends on how much they want to participate in rebalancing their own condition. For myself I find that Shiatsu is the most relaxing yet energizing method of putting me back in touch with *me* – if I could have a Shiatsu treatment every day that would be heaven!

5

How To Give Shiatsu – A Basic Sequence

THE BASIC SEQUENCE which I shall outline below is similar to the one which I teach my beginning students. It is a fairly simple routine designed to stimulate all of the meridians to promote relaxation and ease out many of the everyday aches and pains which we are all prone to from time to time. Being a generalized treatment it is quite appropriate for most people, so once you have mastered it you can practise on your family and friends. It is beyond the scope of this book to go into advanced technique and I would encourage those of you who are fired with curiosity and enthusiasm by doing the basic sequence to go to Shiatsu classes where you can learn further techniques and diagnosis. One of my teachers once advised students to do 500 basic treatments before thinking of going on to more advanced ways of working using hara diagnosis and specific meridians. In many ways I think this is sound advice. By practising the basics until they become second nature you become sufficiently confident not to have to worry about what to do next; at that point you can start to concentrate on how you are working and what you are feeling, and that is the time to start looking at more specific advanced work.

For those of you who do want to take a look at diagnosis I have included a short section on how to do a simplified form of hara diagnosis after the basic sequence. Learning to do proper two-handed hara palpation really requires the presence of an experienced teacher to lead you through the various steps and to help you interpret what you are feeling, but using the simplified form along with the tables of meridian functions and associations (see Chapter 3) can help you to pinpoint any imbalances. You can then concentrate on the relevant meridians within the context of this basic routine to make a 'more specific treatment for a particular condition.

WHEN NOT TO GIVE SHIATSU

Before we start our session there are a few general cautions which we should observe. You should not give Shiatsu in cases of fever, infectious or contagious illnesses, on the site of burns, open sores, broken bones or varicose veins. In the hands of an experienced practitioner Shiatsu can be used for a wide range of health problems but as a beginner you should not tackle any serious or acute complaint, especially cancer, heart disease or any potentially life-threatening condition; it is unwise for a beginner to work on a woman during the first three months of pregnancy, and at all times during pregnancy the points SP6, LI4 and GB21 and heavy pressure below the knee should be avoided because these points may initiate labour or cause miscarriage. In general, work gently round any sites of pain, such as tight or pulled muscles, tendons or tenderness at joints, and if you are in doubt as to whether this basic relaxing treatment is appropriate then take advice from an experienced practitioner.

Complex or serious conditions should be referred to a practitioner registered with the Shiatsu Society (see Chapter 7 for address). As well as the contraindications above, it is common sense not to give Shiatsu within an hour of taking a heavy meal; if your partner is very hungry it is better to let them take a small snack and wait half an hour before starting. Also don't start the session if they are very wound up physically or mentally – give them ten minutes to sit or lie quietly and let breathing and heartbeat come back to normal.

SETTING THE SCENE

Now we are ready to begin. The room you are in is light, airy and above all comfortably warm – your partner will tend to cool down as their metabolism slows so warmth is important. It is good to have a blanket handy to cover hands or feet, especially if they have drifted off to sleep at the end of the session. A pillow is also useful to pad up knees or to put under their chest when lying face downwards to ensure complete relaxation. Remember, relaxation is one of the prime benefits of Shiatsu so your partner should be able to lie comfortably throughout the session. You may want to put on some relaxing music and perhaps burn some aromatic essential oils to enhance the peaceful atmosphere, and of course take steps to prevent interruptions from telephones, children, animals or anything else. This is your partner's quiet time with themselves and everything must be done to allow them to concentrate on that fact.

It is best for both of you to wear loose cotton clothing – a track or jogging suit is ideal as it is warm and allows your partner to stretch into the various positions used in the session. Socks can be worn on the feet if they tend to get cold, but not tights – it is very difficult to stimulate individual toes through tights. From your point of view a jogging suit or other garment that allows you to stretch and move about is essential. I find that I get quite hot as I work and a sweatshirt top is easy to slip off without losing the continuity of the session.

If you have a Japanese futon, that is the ideal surface for giving Shiatsu, but a couple of blankets folded on a carpet is just as comfortable and supportive. Don't give Shiatsu to someone lying on a bed. The effect of the pressure you apply will be lost in the springs, and what is more you will probably end up with a sore back from stooping over. Working on the floor is simpler and much more effective.

ATTITUDE

Your attitude in giving Shiatsu is of paramount importance since you are using your own body and its Ki in order to help another person. This is, in fact, the essence of the spiritual development aspect of Shiatsu – being clear and balanced so as to be most effective. *Calmness* and *concentration* are the key words. You should be in a good mood, not angry, upset, preoccupied or over-tired. Try to clear away any of these negative feelings by breathing deeply into your hara and letting go all negativity as you breathe out. The human mind being what it is, unwanted thoughts like 'what am I going to have for dinner?', 'must remember to phone Auntie Mary', 'am I doing this right?' are bound to pop into your head. Just let them flow through your mind and out again; bring your concentration back to your hands and your partner – rather like in meditation.

Breathing and *centring in hara* are two other important aspects which we have spoken of earlier. As you sit down beside your partner, take a deep breath and let it fill up not just your lungs but the whole of your abdomen right down to the *tanden* (the centre of the hara, three finger-widths below your navel). Relax and breathe right out. This recycles your own Ki and is a good technique to use at the start and finish of a session. During the treatment you can breath in to hara and out through your hands; this has the effect of recycling your Ki so you avoid that unpleasant sensation of being 'drained' by giving out too much. Occasionally too you may come across other unwanted feelings such as heaviness, picking up your partner's negative energy or even getting a headache. Here again the use of breath and also visualization can come into their own. Take a couple of deep breaths into hara to replenish your store of Ki. If your hands are feeling heavy give them a shake, and be sure to breathe out while applying pressure, this helps to ensure that Ki flows from you to your partner, not the other way. At the end of a session I always make a point of washing my hands under cold running water and breathing out a couple of times completely emptying the lungs. This little ritual has the effect of mentally finishing off the treatment, so I am no longer carrying that person or their energy around with me. The mind is a wonderfully powerful tool and can be used in instances like this to make sure that you as well as your partner feel good at the end of the session.

When you apply pressure, keep your *awareness in your hara* at all times and *lean* into the tsubo using relaxed body-weight. This sort of pressure is much less tiring to give and much more comfortable to receive – in fact you will be surprised how hard you can lean on someone when you are centred in hara and they will still find it pleasant. Being grounded in hara also makes you more sensitive to your partner's Ki and you will find it much easier to tune in and give the right quantity and quality of pressure.

PRESSURE

Shiatsu uses the hands, thumbs, elbows, knees and feet to apply pressure to points on the meridians. The most basic of techniques is using the thumb, the palm or the heel of the hand straight into the body at 90 degrees (what is known in the trade as 'perpendicular pressure'). We also generally work with two hands on the body; a *mother hand* which stays still, often resting on the hara or the sacrum, and a *working hand* which is the one to apply active pressure. It is most supportive for your partner if you have two hands on at all times, helping them to connect up different parts of the body and increase their awareness of self.

The pressure should be deep enough to connect with the Ki in the meridian or tsubo you are working on. There is no quantity like 5lbs or 15lbs of pressure which can be prescribed since the appropriate amount of pressure varies with each individual and on different parts of the body. If you stimulate too hard you will hurt your partner causing them to tighten up in order to protect themselves. If your pressure is not sufficiently deep it will feel unsatisfactory to your partner as you won't have connected with the energy. As you concentrate and listen to your hands you will, with practice, start to tune in to your partner's energy intuitively; it will then become easier to be sensitive to the degree of pressure needed. The sensation of connecting with Ki is often accompanied by a sort of 'good pain' for them, while you may feel it as a subtle change of feeling under your thumb. Don't worry if you don't feel this in the first sessions – it takes time to develop sensitivity to Ki, not to mention the confidence to know when you have connected. If you think you are feeling Ki then you probably are! Until you are sure, the best way is to apply pressure on each point for the count of five seconds before moving on to the next point. This gives your thumb or fingers a chance to tune in to the Ki of that tsubo, even though your conscious mind is not aware of connecting with Ki.

As well as the classic deep, straight pressure there are other useful techniques for loosening up tight muscles. Rubbing quickly over the surface with the flat of your hand is good for coldness and superficial tightness. Kneading with thumbs,

71

knuckles or the bony part of the heel of your hand is a good way to start softening up chronically stiff muscles (especially those in the shoulder, upper back, buttock and thigh). Having loosened up you can then work more deeply with thumb or elbow pressure. We always work from general techniques; palming, kneading, rotating, to more specific ones; holding points with thumb, elbow or knees.

A note on the direction of working Different Shiatsu techniques may work the meridians in different directions, for example in Zen Shiatsu the meridians are usually worked from the hara outwards to the extremities, regardless of the Yin or Yang direction of flow. For the purposes of simplicity in this following sequence I have followed the traditional method of working up the Yin meridians and down the Yang, in accordance with the body's natural Ki flow.

REACTIONS TO TREATMENT

Although it is unlikely after a general Shiatsu session such as we are going to learn here, it does sometimes happen that your partner may have what we term a 'healing reaction' after the treatment. This may take the form of a headache, feeling tired or low, or possibly flu-like symptoms, lasting for about 24 hours. Take plenty of spring water and rest to help clear the toxins which have been released, and don't worry unduly. This is the body's way of cleansing itself and is part of the healing process.

THE BASIC SHIATSU SEQUENCE

The Back

Have your partner lie face downwards, head turned to one side (let them know they can move it from side to side to prevent stiffness), hands down towards their sides so that the shoulders are comfortable.

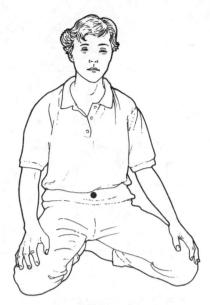

Fig. 7. Sitting in 'seiza' centred at the tanden

1. Sit in seiza (see Figure 7) beside their hips and place one hand on the sacrum (the triangular bone at the base of the spine). Take a couple of deep breaths and centre yourself in hara (in other words just bring your awareness down to the tanden). I call this space of time 'making friends'. It allows you to concentrate your awareness and lets your partner relax and get the feel of your hand. Many people still have reservations about being touched by someone else, so this period is essential to let them relax and open up to receiving.
2. Gently rock the sacrum from side to side by pushing it away from you and letting it roll back, rather like pushing a swing. This is very effective for relaxing the lower back. Take a full minute or more to do this, then let the movement slow down and gently bring it to a stop.
3. Coming up on one knee, place one hand on the sacrum and the other on the opposite side of the spine at the top of the shoulder blade, with the heel of your hand on the band of muscle that runs alongside the spine. The hand on the sacrum is the *mother hand*, listening in to what your partner's body is telling you and giving support. If you stimulate too

73

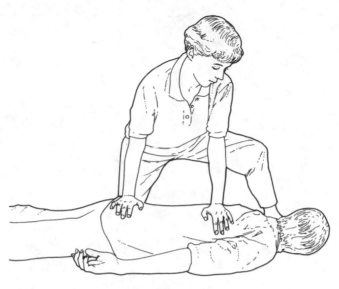

Fig. 8. Palming the back

deeply, mother hand will let you know since the sacrum will react. Breathe out and lean straight down onto your working hand (the one at the shoulder). Breathe in and move it down a palm's width, then breathing out, apply pressure again. (Figure 8.) Remember to move from hara and keep the pressure on for five seconds or so to connect with your partner's Ki. Continue in this way down to the bottom of the buttock. Then take the same hand back up to the other shoulder and stimulate down the other side of the spine in the same way.

Remember, avoid touching the spine, and work more gently over the lumbar (lower back) area where there are no ribs to protect the internal organs. You will find on this, and all the back techniques, that you have to bend your knees and move your hips in order to use your hara effectively to apply pressure. Repeat three times.

4. Now take your mother hand off the sacrum and do a similar technique with both hands, one on each side of the spine. Repeat three times.

5. Take the shoulder muscles one in each hand and make kneading movements to loosen them up.

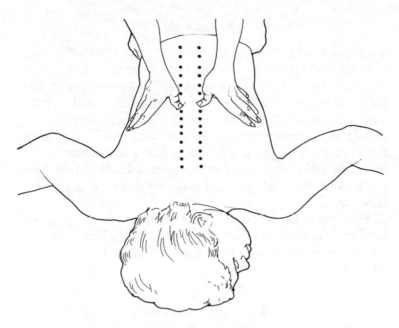

Fig. 9.   Thumbing the BL and Yu Points on the back

6. Starting at a level with the centre of the shoulder blades, place your thumbs one-and-a-half thumbs width out from the spine on both sides and breathing out from hara, lean down onto your thumbs with arms straight. Release (Figure 9). Here we are stimulating the Yu points on the Bladder meridian – check back to Figure 5 for details of which point is related to which meridian and organ. Slide your thumbs down about an inch and press in again; continue on down on either side of the back until you reach the sacrum. Here you work with the thumbs in the *foramen* or notches on the bone, and because the sacrum is a triangular bone your thumbs will tend to come together. Repeat three times.

Remember it is important to move from hara when working on the Yu points as the specific pressure aimed between the lateral processes of the spinal column is connecting directly to the internal organs via the meridian and spinal nerve pathways. Repeat the whole line of Yu points, from the shoulder blades to the tip of the sacrum, three times.

The Buttocks

7. We all tend to hold a lot of tension in our buttocks, some of us also hold stagnation in the form of fat here. Shiatsu can help both these problems. Start by applying pressure with your palms all over the buttocks. Remember to lean in from hara. This will encourage your partner to relax those deep postural muscles where tension can so easily accumulate. Then, placing the heels of both hands into the hollows at the sides of the buttocks, make large circular movements keeping your hand on the same piece of flesh and making the muscle under your hand move.

8. Find the sensitive point in the centre of the buttock and press in three times on each side. This is GB30 – see Figure 11 for the exact location – very good for lower back pain and sciatica.

Leg Yang Meridians

9. Move down to beside the legs. Place the mother hand on the sacrum and with your working hand, palm down the middle of the back of the leg from thigh to ankle. Avoid pressure on the back of the knee as it is uncomfortable on the kneecap. Next thumb down the same line three times – this is still the Bladder meridian (Figure 10). Be sensitive on the calf muscle as this is often sore. At the Achilles tendon, pinch the tendon between thumb and index finger, then pinch down the outside of the foot to the little toe.

10. Bend the foot up towards the buttock and slide the knee outwards so that the side of the leg is exposed. This is the stretch position for the Gall bladder meridian which runs down the side of the leg to the fourth toe. Using the same sequence as for Bladder, palm down Gall bladder then thumb it three times. Mother hand should still be on the sacrum (Figure 11).

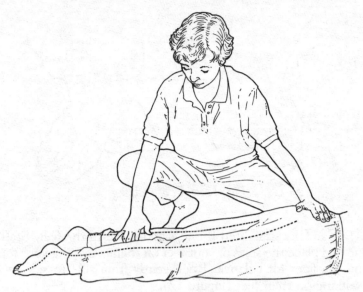

Fig. 10.   Thumbing the Bladder meridian in the leg

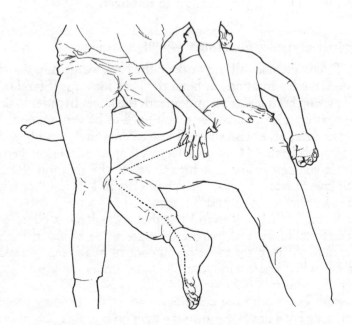

Fig. 11.   Thumbing GB30 and Gall bladder meridian

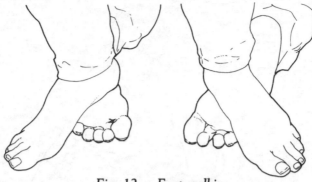

Fig. 12. Foot walking

11. Carefully straighten the legs and move to the feet. Stand up and place the soles of your feet on theirs, keeping your toes on the floor for balance. Rock gently from side to side as if walking on their feet (Figure 12).

Now move over to the other side of the body and repeat the Bladder and Gall bladder meridians on this side, that is parts 9 to 11. Ask your partner to roll over.

Leg rotations

12. To complement all the work on the back we are now going to do some leg rotations to bend the back forwards. Stand up and pick up both legs from underneath the knee. In order to do the next couple of movements you have to be very grounded in your hara, otherwise you will lose balance and possibly end up with backache. Have your feet well apart and knees bent so that you can swing your hips to create the rotation. Push both knees up to your partner's chest (Figure 13), hold for ten seconds, release, then push in again.

13. Swing both knees round together in as large a circle as is comfortable for your partner. Rotate three times in each direction. A little tip to help you control heavy legs – hold just below the knees with your hands just under the kneecaps, as in the illustration.

14. Push knees onto the chest again and then, keeping them bent, take both knees down to the floor on one side, and then the other. This creates a nice twist on the lower back.

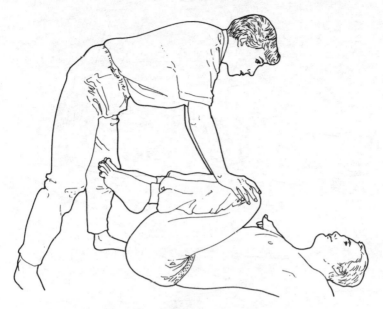

Fig. 13. Two knees to chest

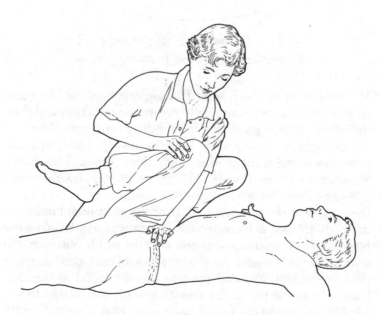

Fig. 14. Single leg rotation

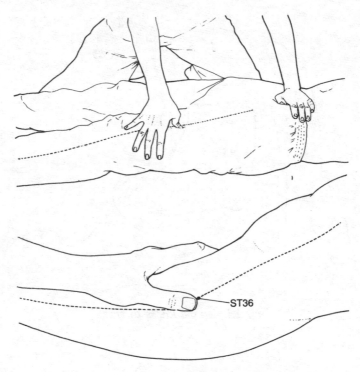

Fig. 15. Stomach meridian at front of leg
Detail showing position position of ST36

15. Straighten out both legs. Placing one hand on the hara, pick up one leg and rotate it slowly in one direction and then the other. This is good for hip mobilization (Figure 14).
16. Straighten the leg and, keeping mother hand on hara, palm down the front of the thigh three times. This is the Stomach meridian (Figure 15). Now thumb straight down this same line. Below the knee the Stomach meridian runs to the outside of the shin bone. One of the most useful points in the body (ST36) is located here four fingers-width below the bottom of the kneecap and one thumbs-width out from the shin bone; it is useful for digestive problems, tiredness and pain in the legs. Press all the way down parallel to the shin bone, across the top of the foot to end on the second toe.
17. Move down to the foot. Cradle it on your knee and rotate the ankle in both directions as far as it will comfortably go. Squeeze down the top and sole of the foot, and with a loose fist lightly tap all over the sole. Press KD1 which is found in

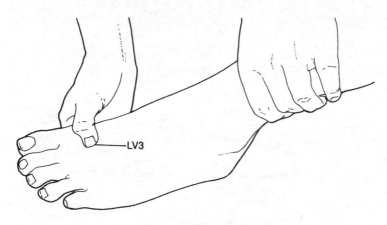

Fig. 16. Position of LV3

the centre of the foot just below the ball – Figure 18 shows the exact location. Now work on LV3 in the hollow on the top of the foot just behind the big toe (Figure 16). Rotate each toe in turn, squeeze and pull down the sides of each toe to stimulate the beginnings and endings of the meridians.

Leg Yin Meridians

18. Move back to beside the hips, pick up the leg, rotate and place it with the knee bent outwards and the instep beside the opposite ankle. This is the stretch position for the Spleen meridian, which runs from the outside of the big toe round the top of the ankle, up the inside of the shin bone and on to the inside of the front thigh (Figure 17). On the way up, the meridian passes through SP6 (three fingers-width above the inner ankle bone, and just behind the bone) whose oriental name means 'three yin meeting point' since Spleen, Liver and Kidney meridians all meet in this point. SP6 is very effective for any kind of menstrual and gynaecological problem, and also for pain in the lower body. *SP6 should not be used during pregnancy as heavy stimulation here can cause miscarriage.* Thumb three times from the outside of the big toe to SP6 and then along the inside of the shin (keeping just behind the bone) to the knee. Above the knee, palm the meridian twice and then move to more specific pressure. This is a nice area in which to use your elbows as they can give strong, relaxed pressure through the

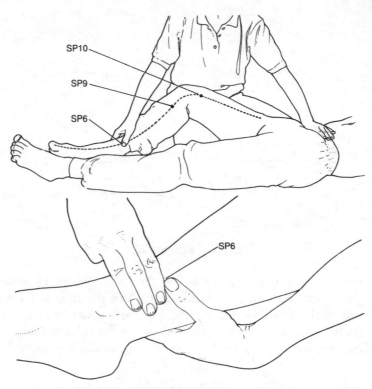

Fig. 17. Spleen/Pancreas meridian
Detail showing position of SP6 – three finger widths above the inner ankle

large thigh muscles. As you can see from the illustration, the meridian runs just to the inside of the front thigh. Remember to keep mother hand on the hara to listen in to what the Ki is doing. Repeat this upper part three times.

19. Pick up the leg from the knee, as before, rotate several times and then place with the instep to the knee. This is the stretch position for the Liver meridian, which runs from the inside of the big toe, between the first and second toes up to the front of the ankle and up into SP6. From there it continues up the front of the lower leg, actually on the bone, until two-thirds of the way up the shin, where it sweeps back crossing over Spleen, runs through the inside of the knee and up the thigh parallel to Spleen but immediately behind the adductor longus muscle (the inside thigh muscle which tends

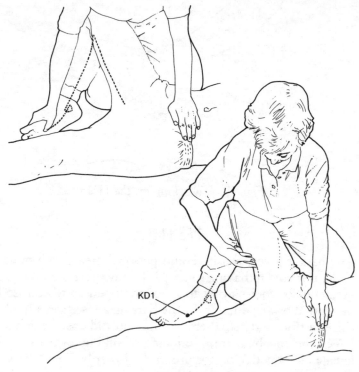

Fig. 18. Kidney meridian
Detail showing position of KD1

to be tight in many people). Work the Liver meridian in the same way as Spleen. Thumb the lower leg, then palm and thumb or elbow the thigh three times.

20. The third of this trio of leg yin meridians is the Kidney meridian. Its stretch position is with the foot placed as high as possible, as in Figure 18. Start at KD1, 'Bubbling Spring', on the sole of the foot just below the ball, and work with thumb pressure round the base of the inside ankle, through SP6 and further round onto the calf muscle as far as the knee. Above the knee, work with palm or fingertips, as in the picture, quite far round towards the back of the upper leg.

21. Rotate the leg again and carefully straighten it. Move over to the other side and work through parts 15 to 21 again, so that both legs are evenly stimulated. Now move up to level with the hara.

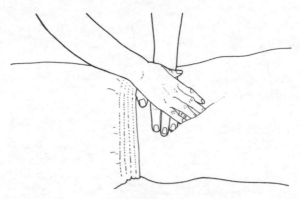

Fig. 19. Working on the Hara

The Hara

The hara is a very sensitive and personal area which most of us are not used to having touched. It may therefore take a few moments for your partner to relax and open up to you, so be patient. Working directly on the hara means we can stimulate the intestines and help them to eliminate old waste which may have been caught there, producing a build up of toxins. The female reproductive organs are in the lower hara and working here can help with menstrual problems as well as preventing the build up of waste and toxins in the ovaries and uterus. If your partner is a woman, ask if she has a period and work very gently if this is the case.

22. Sit so that you are facing your partner. Place one hand on top of the other on the centre of the hara and take a couple of moments to 'make friends' again. Start slowly rocking back and forwards with your body and at the same time make a push-pull action with your hands, rather like kneading dough very slowly. This is not a rubbing action – your hands should be in contact with the same bit of flesh, but making a firm, wave-like motion to move the intestines under your hands. Keep this up for three full minutes, starting fairly lightly, working more deeply and then coming up again and gently to rest. Don't stop suddenly as this can be disconcerting for your partner.

23. Now turn sideways to sit parallel and place your further-away hand over the tanden. Starting at the solar plexus, with

your working hand you are going to stimulate right round the outside edge of the hara. If you imagine that their hara is a clock face, you are going to press in on each number right around the clock. Lean straight down with your fingertips as you both breathe out (Figure 19). Breathe in and move your working hand round to the next position, breathe out again. Continue in a steady rhythm twice round the hara, then using the same technique take a line down the centre of the hara. Do not press directly on the navel.

The Chest

Emotional problems, breathing difficulties, lung and heart conditions all 'stick' in the chest.

24. Place your thumbs in the spaces between the ribs at the base of the ribcage. Holding each point for five seconds, proceed up the ribcage stimulating into each space close in to the sternum. Avoid pressing on breast tissue. When you reach the underside of the collarbone, follow its line out until you reach the tender hollow just before the shoulder joint. One thumbs-width down from that hollow is LU1, very good for any lung problem, chestiness or a tickly cough (Figure 20).

25. Place your nearside hand on your partner's shoulder and hold the wrist with your other hand. Now, supporting the shoulder joint firmly, make a large slow rotation, rather like

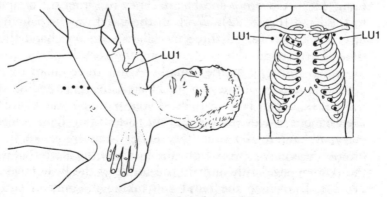

Fig. 20. Thumbing LU1
Detail showing points on Lung meridian – points between ribs to be worked up the chest

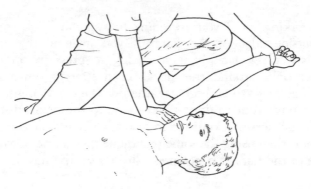

Fig. 21. Arm rotation

swimming the back-stroke. Stretch the arm up (Figure 21), then out to the side, then pull down and stretch both arm and shoulder towards the feet. Once you get the hang of it, this is a lovely, fluid stretch which really eases out the shoulder and chest muscles.

Arm Yin Meridians

26. Lay the arm out straight to the side with palm uppermost. Now we have the three yin meridians of the arm exposed: Lung, Heart Governor and Heart. They run from the armpit to the hand (Figure 22). Work in the usual way by palming first; you can cover all three meridians with one hand this time. Then thumb three times along the topside of the arm for Lung, finishing at the thumb. Again three times right down the middle of the arm for Heart Governor, ending at the middle finger. For Heart bend your partner's arm so that their hand is above their head; if they are stiff in the shoulder you may have to slip your knee under their elbow. In this position it is easy to work from the inside of the armpit along the bottom edge of the arm to the inside of the little finger.
27. Move down to the hand and taking it firmly in both of yours spread the palm open wide with sweeping thumb movements. Then knead over the whole of the palm, rotate each finger in turn, squeeze down the sides of the fingers and give each a little pull. This stimulates the beginnings and endings of the arm meridians. The hand has several useful

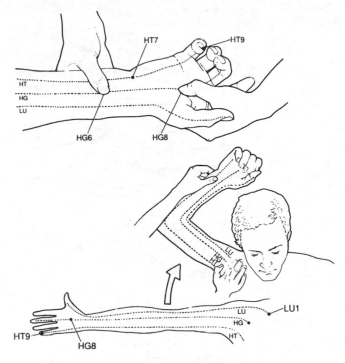

Fig. 22. Arm yin meridians
HT stretch and hand and wrist points

points: HG8 in the centre of the palm for heart-related pain and anxiety; HT9 on the inside of the little finger, also good for heart problems and palpitations; LI4 on the back of the hand between thumb and index finger. *Do not use LI4 during pregnancy as it may cause miscarriage or early labour.* LI4 is good for intestinal problems, headache and general vitality. Press for ten seconds three times with your thumb, using your index finger to support on the palm. For most people this is a tender point, so be sensitive and use your hara.

Arm Yang Meridians

28. Place the arm palm downwards so as to expose the Large Intestine, Triple Heater and Small Intestine meridians. They run from the fingers down the back of the arm to the shoulder,

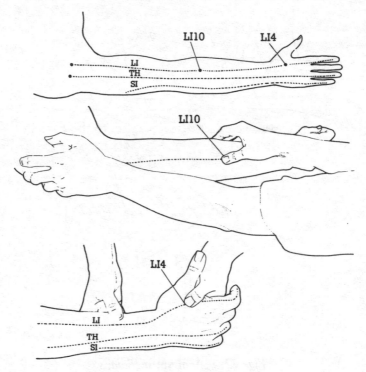

Fig. 23. *Arm yang meridians*
Detail showing position of LI10
near elbow and on hand LI4

and then on to the head. Remember, our meridian man was standing with his arms up to the sky to receive Yang from Heaven and Yin from the Earth; so the flow of Yang in the arm meridians runs from hands to shoulder. Palm all three meridians at once, with mother hand on the shoulder. Then thumb Large Intestine from the end of the index finger, through LI4, in the web between index finger and thumb, and LI10, a tsubo on the top of the forearm muscle three fingers-width down from the inside elbow crease (Figure 23). LI10 is good for waking you up and energizing, also a useful point for pain control in the arms and upper body. Continue thumbing between the biceps and triceps to the front dimple on top of the deltoid muscle – if you can't feel it ask your partner to abduct their arm upwards, and you will feel the two dimples at the top of the muscle quite clearly.

29. Now thumb Triple Heater meridian from the ring finger, between the bones of the forearm and along the back of the upper arm to the back dimple on the top of the deltoid muscle.

30. Small Intestine runs from the outside of the little finger close along the back of the ulna bone, then along the middle of the triceps on the back of the upper arm to the back of the armpit crease. You can thumb it in this position, or place the arm across the chest to get into the upper part a little more easily. As usual, work three times. Give the arm a shake and lay it down. Move over to the other arm and repeat parts 25 to 30.

Neck and Head

31. Now move up so that you are sitting above your partner's head. Push their shoulders down and away from you to stretch the neck, then slip your hands under their neck and pull the head gently towards you by leaning back. Alternate this push-pull three or four times.

32. With your fingertips underneath the neck, work in small circles to loosen the muscles on the back of the neck, all the way up to the base of the skull. Then press in on either side of the spine up the length of the neck. The pressing technique here is actually placing your fingers and pulling towards yourself gently by leaning back. Remember that your pressure should go into the body at ninety degrees. When you reach the head work into any tight points along the base of the skull.

33. Turn the head to one side and stimulate GB20 which is found in the hollow between the two large neck muscles – trapezius and sternocleidomastoid (Figure 24). Headaches, neck tension and pain, and stiffness can all be treated by working GB20. Gently thumb down the side of the neck along the top of the shoulder muscle until you meet the bones of the shoulder joint. Turn the head and work the other side.

34. Centre the head. Remember that all pressure on your partner's head should be firm but gentle. Putting one thumb on top of the other, work from between the eyebrows up the centre of the forehead to the top of the crown (Figure 25).

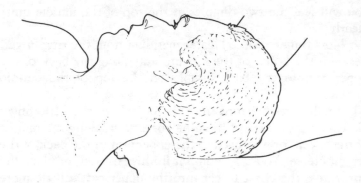

Fig. 24. Position of GB20

Come back to the eyebrows and slide your index fingers down into the little notch at the upper inside corner of the eye socket; pull back to apply pressure. This is BL2, good for relieving headaches and eye strain.

35. Now follow the line of the eye socket right round, applying pressure with your fingers at the top and your thumbs on the lower border. Make sure you don't drag the skin here as it is delicate – this is Shiatsu for facial beauty!

36. Make gentle circles at the temples. Slide your index fingers down either side of the nose to LI20 at the outer corner of the nostril. LI20 helps to relieve nasal congestion. Next work outwards along the bottom of the cheekbones, pressing slightly upwards under the bone. When you reach the jaw muscle

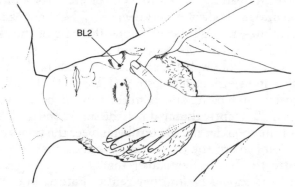

*Fig. 25. Working GV on the forehead
and showing position of BL2*

make slow but firm circling movements as this area tends to be very tight, especially in people who suppress their anger. With gentle pressure work around the lips over the teeth and gum areas, then squeeze along the lower jaw with thumb and index finger.

37. Finally, using your index finger and thumb, massage all over the ears, and pull the ear lobes down towards the shoulders. Very soothing!

38. Move back to sit beside your partner's hara and place a hand on the tanden, just below the navel. Take three deep, slow breaths into your own hara, allowing warm, positive, healing Ki to flow from your hand to your partner. Let your hand rest there for a moment or two as you mentally 'finish off' the session. Then quietly move away, cover them with a blanket if it seems appropriate, and go and wash your hands. You should also make a point of taking three or four deep breaths to recharge yourself in case you have expended too much of your own Ki in the course of the session.

Written out like this a basic session seems very long, but as you practise you will get quicker, so that you can easily go through all this in about an hour. In fact your sessions should never be much longer than an hour. Certainly not if your partner has a weak condition, since too much manipulation of their energy will tend to dissipate it. A short session using just part of this sequence, say the back or hands and feet, can be very relaxing and revitalizing. My purpose in showing you the whole of a basic session is that, once you have mastered it and are familiar with it, you can choose to concentrate on some parts, skip over others, improvise, add more techniques – in short, be creative. Shiatsu is not a fixed routine in which techniques follow each other in a special order; each session should be a unique and creative event. Using a 'form' like this basic session helps us to learn the basic techniques of Shiatsu in a logical and easy-to-remember framework; it also means that you have a range of techniques to cover all of the body. Once you have become proficient in the form you can focus more on what you are feeling with your hands, and so choose the appropriate techniques for your partner's needs at the time.

In professional practice a therapist may have their own personal order of working, or may rely upon their intuition to guide them as to which areas to concentrate upon on that occasion. Personally I always start with hara diagnosis, unless the patient is new to me and extremely nervous, in which case I would work first on their back. Having taken a reading from hara and discovered which meridians are most out of balance, I would then work the relevant meridians (usually two, occasionally three) in either the legs or the arms first, including hands and feet which I invariably cover in order to stimulate the beginnings and ends of all the meridians, and then the same meridians in whichever limb I had not already covered.

For example, on a diagnosis of Heart Governor kyo and Bladder jitsu, I would tonify Heart Governor in the chest and arm and possibly sedate the supplementary Bladder meridian in the arm. I would then tonify supplementary Heart Governor in the leg before turning over and working the back, essentially Bladder, and the back of the leg in a sedating fashion. The back with the Yu points is an essential part of treatment which I never miss out, and I generally end with the neck and a relaxing massage on the face. Sometimes I would then move to their feet to 'ground' them before returning to hara for another hara diagnosis to tell me what had shifted in the session. I also use a more subtle etheric technique to read and balance the Three Heaters, the three central chakras, situated at the heart, solar plexus and tanden. For me each session is very different, and even with a similar diagnosis coming up, each person requires a different approach and application of techniques. This is what is so fascinating about giving Shiatsu.

SIMPLE ONE-HANDED HARA DIAGNOSIS

Once you have become accustomed to giving the basic Shiatsu sequence laid out in this chapter, you may want to start homing in on particular meridians to help rebalance certain health conditions. By using the table of meridian associations and imbalances in Chapter 3 and the simplified form of hara diagnosis that follows, we can make a reasonably accurate diagnosis using the kyo-jitsu model, which can then be applied to your basic sequence by simply concentrating more on the specified meridians and leaving out other parts of the form. I would stress that this is not a full Shiatsu diagnosis and if you want to learn properly you should arrange to go to Shiatsu classes. You cannot really learn any hands-on practical skill in any depth from a book – much better to have a qualified person by your side to guide you.

Look back to Figure 4 (page 47) which shows Masunaga's map of the hara diagnostic areas. Sit in seiza beside your partner facing their head with your thigh making contact with the side of their body. Using a *relaxed* hand and fairly light touch, feel each of the areas in turn with the hand nearest your partner to see how far your fingertips sink into their hara at each position. The secret here is to keep your fingers very loose and angle them so that you are going straight in at 90 degrees. Imagine you are dipping your fingertips slowly into a bowl of water to see how hot it is. What we are feeling for is kyo or jitsu quality: does the area feel loose or tight, yielding or resistant, soft or bouncy? Rather than pressing in, try to rest your fingers on the surface of the hara and note how far the hara allows you to sink in. If there is no resistance or reaction or if it feels very soft, that is a kyo feeling. Jitsu feels firmer or bouncy and definitely responds to your touch.

Now go through all the areas again in the same way and try to pinpoint which area feels the most kyo and which the most jitsu. The order which we generally use to go through the hara areas is HT, GB, LV, right LU, ST, TH, left LU, HT, HG, SP (use the flat of your fingers so as not to pick up the pulse), KD, BL, left LI, left SI, right LI, right SI. By going round the areas in the same order (which is, by the way, merely a convention) we get into a routine which allows us to concentrate on *what* we are feeling, not where we are going next or whether we have missed out any of the areas.

Having found a most kyo and a most jitsu diagnostic area, these correspond to the meridians most out of balance and therefore you can give them more attention in your session. Usually we spend more time on tonifying the kyo as this is seen as the cause of imbalance. Over a period of time if you work on someone regularly you will start to see patterns emerging in diagnosis which, if you note them and look up their theoretical associations, will show you how theory and practice correlate and work together in concert. This is the real start of your journey of understanding into the fascinating world of the workings of Ki.

6

Related Exercises and Self-Help Measures

BY NOW YOU will see that giving Shiatsu is not just about applying a set of techniques to a body; it is a whole way of living and being. The perceptions and sensitivity we use in Shiatsu are innate qualities which we can develop with practice and through particular exercises. Many of these are very simple, take little time to do and can very easily be incorporated into everyday life. Students of Shiatsu are taught self-development exercises to help them in their practice, and I often give some of these exercises to my patients as 'homework' to help them with a particular problem.

The important thing about exercises is that they have to be within the grasp of the person doing them. It is no good expecting the overweight and 'pushed for time' businessman to go jogging for an hour every lunchtime, any more than it is any good expecting a night bird like me to get up and do an hour's yoga before breakfast!

Personally, I especially like exercises and self-help measures that I can do either relatively quickly or even while carrying on with the rest of the day's business. This is not to say that I have never taken time on my personal development practices; there was a period in my life when I spent considerable time in meditation, yoga, aikido, cooking perfectly Yin-Yang balanced meals and other pursuits. These days with a busy practice and Shiatsu school to run, not to mention looking after my family and being involved in work with charities, I find that my work and the principles I use in it are my self-development exercises. For me, practising Shiatsu for six or more hours per day is sufficient spiritual and physical discipline. However, I am in a privileged position; if you are just starting out on the road of Shiatsu and self understanding, try to take at least half an hour every day on some of these exercises. Spending time alone, just being with ourselves, is important for all of us, to remind us of who we are, especially those who have heavy demands made of them. As a busy mother said to me recently: 'Being by myself and doing something positive for me makes me feel like *me* again!'

When people first come to Shiatsu I feel they need activities that will not take too much time, but will be effective. The following exercises are ones that are simple and can really make a difference to the quality of your life.

HARA DEVELOPMENT AND
BREATHING EXERCISES

One of the most powerful things we can learn in life is how to be in touch with our hara. In the orient it is said that mind and body come together in the hara: here is the centre of our physical energy and our mental forces – the very essence of our Self. The first step to being able to harness the power of hara is awareness.

Exercise 1

Place your fingertips on the tanden, the centre of your hara, three fingers-width below the navel, and press in. Imagine a ball of light there deep inside your body. On and off during the day, remember about this ball of light and just be aware of it as you go about your normal activities. Next time you have to climb a lot of stairs or run for any length of time, instead of thinking about your tired legs or sore chest, think of the ball of light in your hara; you will find it easier to get to where you want to be. Using hara is also effective in emotional situations: if you feel yourself becoming angry or frightened take several deep breaths, allowing the breath to expand right down to your hara, be conscious of your tanden, if necessary you can even touch it to centre yourself. Your anger or fear will now be more controlled and you will feel more distanced from the situation and able to react appropriately.

Exercise 2

This is one to do quietly for ten minutes by yourself. Sit comfortably with your spine straight, either on a chair or on the floor crosslegged or in seiza. Become aware of your hara. As you breathe in through your nose, imagine your breath as a stream of light filling up your hara. Keep the image of light at the hara and let the excess breath slip out through your mouth, so that you create a reservoir of light in your hara that grows stronger with every in-breath. This can be done as an exercise on its own or as a preparation for giving Shiatsu. If you are about to give Shiatsu, you can then extend the exercise by breathing out the stream of light through your hands and into your partner. The light is of course a visualization of Ki.

Exercise 3

Again taking a quiet few minutes to yourself, breath to hara as in the last exercise. Then instead of filling up the hara, fill up the whole of your body with light and Ki with each deep inhalation, and exhaling empty the light out until only a little ball remains at your tanden. This is a good exercise if you have been feeling drained or negative, because it allows you to visualize emptying out all the old stale Ki and bringing in new positive energy.

Exercise 4

This exercise concentrates more on breathing. It has a calming effect. I call it 'breathing a square' because you breathe in to the count of four (as fast or slowly as is comfortable), hold your breath for four, breathe out to the count of four and again hold for four. As you do this, be aware of your hara and be careful not to let your shoulders come up as you hold the breath. Let the Ki settle down in hara as you hold your breath.

There are lots of other breathing and hara exercises which you may learn if you go to Shiatsu classes; the ones described above are easy ones which you can start with simply and safely on your own.

STIMULATION OF THE MERIDIANS

Do-In or self-Shiatsu is an energizing routine which can be used at any time of day. There are several different versions with lots of variations but the one which I like is an invigorating tapping routine following the meridians.

Facial Do-In

Start by tapping with your fingers on the top of your head. If you keep a loose wrist you can tap quite hard – it helps to wake up the brain in the morning! Then smoothe across your forehead, followed by circles at your temples with fingertips. Squeeze along your eyebrows. As in the facial Shiatsu routine, stimulate points around your eye socket, being careful not to drag the skin. Rub your cheeks and the end of your nose – both good for the circulation. Press into LI20 at the bottom outside corner of the nostrils and then work with thumbs under your cheekbones out as far as your ears – this helps nasal congestion and sinus problems. Pull your ears up, down, back and forward, and rub all over – again, good for circulation. Pinch along the lower jaw, allowing your thumbs to linger on any little nodules, lymph glands, to squeeze out the toxins.

Neck and shoulders

Going as far as you can comfortably, rotate your head in a circle slowly one way and then the other. If any position is sore then place your hand on your head and gently stretch the neck in that place using the weight of your hand to pull down. Making a loose fist, tap on each shoulder in turn. Shoulders often hold a lot of tension, and a good pounding here can release long-held stress.

Chest and arms

Next tap all over your chest (though avoid breast tissue if you are a woman); this can loosen up mucus and make you cough it up. For even greater effect do it with a 'Tarzan' yell! Continue tapping on the arms: up the Yin meridians on the inner arm from shoulder to hand, turn your arm over and come back down the Yang meridians from hand to shoulder. Squeeze and pull each finger in turn and stimulate LI4 and HG8 (look back to Chapter 5 or further on in this chapter for the exact locations).

Back and legs

Bend forwards and, starting as high up on the back as you can, pummel down either side of the spine from shoulderblade to buttocks. Again you can give yourself a good thump if you keep a loose wrist – this stimulates the Bladder meridian. Now pound away on the buttocks to disperse those extra ounces. Continuing to tap with a loose fist, work down the outsides of the legs, and up the insides – as always going with the Yin-Yang flow. Sit down. Rub the top of your foot, tap all over the sole, and then squeeze and pull each toe in turn. Press in on KD1.

HARA MASSAGE

Lie down with your knees bent up. Lacing your fingers together, rock your hara from side to side in the same way as we did in the Shiatsu sequence. Remember not to rub, but to let the intestines move under your hands. Do this for several minutes. Now starting at the top of the hara at the solar plexus, press inward with your outstretched fingers as you breathe out. Breathe in and move your fingers round to your left (following the direction of digestion), press in again as you exhale. Continue right round the hara just inside the ribs and pelvis, for one and a half circuits. Finally lay your hands over the tanden and rest for several minutes.

THE MAKKO-HO STRETCHES

The Makko-ho stretches are a series of meridian opening movements which are practised widely by Shiatsu practitioners and students. They are useful not just because they stretch each pair of meridians, but because you can monitor the state of your own meridians by the ease and flexibility with which you can get into each position. Some of the poses are similar to ones used in yoga, but the way of working into them is different. With the Makko-ho exercises the attitude is a relaxed one: take a breath in, move into the stretch as you breathe out and relax. Staying in position, breathe in and as you exhale try to relax a little further down into the stretch. Don't bounce or try to push yourself into the pose, just go down as far as is comfortable. We usually do three long exhalations for each stretch, and the order in which they are done is in accordance with the time of day cycle (see Chapter 3).

Lung/Large Intestine (Figure 26)

Stand with feet hip-width apart, link your thumbs behind your back and bending down stretch your arms as far up as possible. Breathe in and out three times trying to relax down on each exhalation.

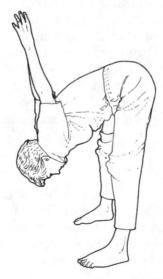

Fig. 26.   Lung/Large Intestine Makko-ho stretch

Stomach/Spleen (Figure 27)

Kneel down with your bottom between your feet, breathe out and lean back onto your elbows. If this is comfortable, on

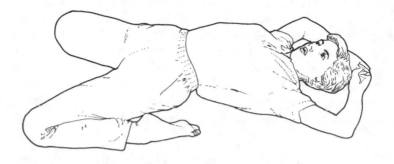

Fig. 27. Stomach/Spleen Makko-ho stretch

the next exhalation go right down to the floor and raise your hands over your head. Breathe in and out three times. Come up in the same stages, grasping your ankles, tucking chin to chest and pushing up strongly on your elbows to bring your back off the floor. Then bend forward to counteract the back bend. If this is too difficult here is a modified version. Sit in seiza, place your hands behind you, breathe out and raise your hips. Hold for three long breaths. This also creates a stretch on the Stomach and Spleen meridians in the front of the thigh.

Heart/Small Intestine (Figure 28)

Sit with the soles of your feet together, drawn up as close to your groin as possible. Clasp your feet, elbows outside your shins, and relax down towards the floor, trying to keep chest and hara open. Again hold the position for three breaths and relaxing down a little on each exhalation.

Bladder/Kidney (Figure 29)

Feet straight out in front of you, bend forward from the hips and push your hands (little fingers uppermost) between your feet if you can reach. If you can't reach your feet then hold your ankles or shins just as far as you can go. Breathe and

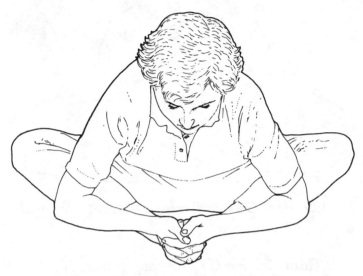

Fig. 28.   Heart/Small Intestine Makko-ho stretch

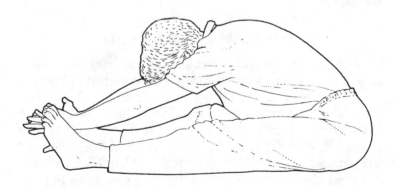

Fig. 29.   Bladder/Kidney Makko-ho stretch

relax down. For the first two breaths look forward between your feet; for the final one tuck your head down towards your knees to stretch the back of the neck.

101

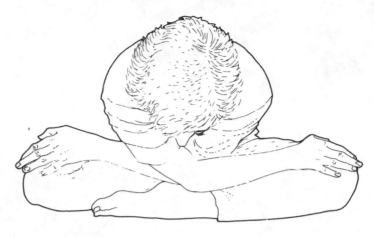

Fig. 30. Heart Governor/Triple Heater Makko-ho stretch

Heart Governor/Triple Heater (Figure 30)

Sit crosslegged and cross your arms the other way clasping your knees. Breathe out and stretch forward pushing your knees down. Again three breaths, then reverse legs and arms and repeat.

Gall bladder/Liver (Figure 31)

Sit with your legs as wide apart as possible. Imagine you have your back to a wall; with your right arm stretched up and your left on your side, stretch down to the left as if sliding down the wall and trying to touch the floor behind your left foot. Hold for three breaths. Come up and reverse arms, slide over to your right in the same way. Remember to keep your back straight and don't collapse your hara. Come back to centre and then clasping your hands in front of you, bend from the hips straight to the front. Again take three long breaths as you relax into the stretch.

That is the full round. Although these stretches take no more than five minutes to do, they are a most effective way of keeping you fit and supple, not to mention helping you feel how each pair of meridians is acting in your body. The Makkoho exercises can be done every morning and

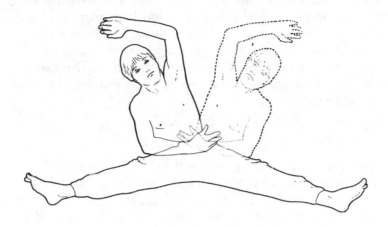

Fig. 31. Gall bladder/Liver Makko-ho stretch

night. Remember, however, that you will be more stiff in the
morning and work accordingly.

MEDITATION

Exercises to calm the mind are just as important as physical
exercises in Shiatsu. Meditation is the traditional way of
stilling the mind and bringing it under control, leading to a
sense of peace, well-being and self understanding. There are
many schools and methods of meditation all of which have
great value. When we start on the path of self development
many of us find that the mind will not be still enough by itself,
and therefore the two meditation exercises I have included
here are ones in which you have to do something.

Exercise 1

Find an object from nature; a stone or a leaf, or a plant, and
place it in front of you. Take five or so minutes to observe it,
pick it up, turn it over, feel it. Place it down again and

imagine where it came from: how the seed came to grow to the plant, or how the pebble was ground down from a great rock. Look at all the small details on it. If other thoughts about other things come into your mind, just let them float away again as you bring your attention back to your object. Do this exercise every day for a week with the same object, then choose a different one. It is amazing that as adults we often forget the wonder of small things in nature. This exercise can bring back that sense of wonder while focusing our mind at the same time.

Exercise 2

Find a quiet place where you will be undisturbed for five or ten minutes. This is a 'Heaven and Earth meditation' which I often do as a guided visualization for my students. Close your eyes and see yourself in your mind's eye in the room where you are sitting comfortably. Imagine yourself floating to the top of the room, and then out into the air above the building. Very slowly float upwards so that you can see the rooftops and trees, then higher and higher until you become aware of the larger geographical features, hills, lakes, rivers, perhaps the sea. Continue up higher until you can see the whole country lying beneath you and the ocean. Then become aware of the continents and as you go even higher, of the Earth as a planet. Finally rest out in space looking back at the beautiful green and blue sphere which is our Earth. How far away and precious it looks. You cannot see any wars or disasters or your own troubles; just a beautiful round wholeness. Now slowly come back through the atmosphere towards your country. As you draw nearer to the Earth, notice the seas, then the hills, rivers, towns, houses, trees. Back you come to above the building where you began, down into the room where you are sitting. Take a deep breath, in and out. Now you are going to imagine yourself feeling very heavy, so heavy that you sink down through the floor into the ground. Sink down into the moist earth and see the roots of plants and trees, the tunnels of mice and moles, stones, maybe old buried ruins. Down you sink through a layer of rock, coming out into a subterranean cavern with a river running through, stalagmites and stalactites decorate the floor and ceiling. Go down even further and you reach a cave where crystals twinkle. It feels warm and safe here, as if you are held in the arms of the mother Earth. Now slowly retrace your steps up through the layers of rock, the stones and streams, up through the fertile earth where the roots of plants feed, back up to the light and your own room. Bring yourself back into awareness of yourself sitting in your chair, in this time and place. Slowly stretch and move a little, and when you feel quite ready, open your eyes.

That is one of my favourite guided meditations. It gives a sense of perspective and connectedness with the Earth and our place on it. Once you have done it a few times you can actually take yourself on that trip quite swiftly and I find it has a very centring effect in times of stress.

FOOD

'You are what you eat' we are told frequently, and certainly commonsense tells us that it is so. What most of us are not so aware of are the more subtle energetic effects that food can have on our health, our moods, our overall state of Ki. There are so many different dietary regimes that we may be forgiven for wondering what it is best to eat, and indeed, with pollution, irradiation and chemicals all part of modern day living, asking if it is safe to eat anything at all!

There is no definitive answer. The traditional oriental view of diet looks for a balance of the 'five tastes' (bitter, sweet, spicy, salty, sour) from the Five Element correspondences, and a balance of Yin or Yang foods according to the time of year and the needs of the individual. Macrobiotics is a modern derivation of traditional Japanese diet, and classifies food and cooking methods by the Yin Yang principle: Yang foods growing below or on the ground, Yin foods above the ground or on bushes and trees. Yang cooking is slower, with pressure or in an oven and with salt; Yin methods include steaming, and raw food. Some people find the guidelines provided by Macrobiotics immensely useful, especially in cases of illness; others find them too restricting.

Personally I feel that whatever dietary regime you follow, food should be a pleasure, not a source of stress or guilt. We should eat in order to live, not the other way around. Each of us must find out our ideal diet and let it work positively for us. There is not space in this book to go into detail about good nutrition, however most dietary therapists and nutritionists would agree with the following simple guidelines to ensure good health.

1. Make sure that you eat regularly, chewing your food properly, and don't eat if you are feeling particularly stressed or angry.

2. Eat plenty of fruit and vegetables – ideally organic if you have a source, or home grown. Two portions of vegetables (either cooked or raw) and at least one piece of fruit per day is a rough guide.

3. Make sure you take enough protein: beans, tofu, fish (not farmed), eggs (free range). If you eat red meat try to restrict it to once or twice per week. Some people like to eat their protein separately from carbohydrate, as this can make digestion easier.

4. Increase your intake of whole grains, such as brown rice, millet, buckwheat, oats and barley. Other good sources of fibre are wholemeal pasta, couscous, nuts and seeds.

5. Many people do not digest bread very well, either because of wheat allergy, or the yeast used. Personally if I eat bread I get a stuffed-up nose immediately, so I only use it as 'emergency food'. Other people find it causes intestinal gas which can be very uncomfortable. Substitute oatcakes, ricecakes, or rye crispbreads instead if you find you cannot take bread.

6. Stimulants such as tea, coffee, chocolate, sugar and the chemicals found in processed and packeted food are in general not beneficial for our health. Herb teas, coffee substitutes, pure fruit juices and plain spring water are the best drinks, but if you are very attached to your stimulating 'cuppa' then allow yourself just one or two per day. A note of caution if you are a heavy coffee drinker; wean yourself off it slowly as sudden withdrawal can cause very unpleasant symptoms. Sugar can be just as addictive; try a little honey in drinks and dried fruit to sweeten desserts instead. In the long run giving up sugar can be the most beneficial, health-promoting measure you could make in your diet.

7. Some people have problems digesting dairy products as they can lead to an overproduction of mucus, resulting in sinus

trouble, digestive and skin complaints. Children are often sensitive to milk and in cases of eczema and asthma you could try cutting out milk for a couple of months as this may help considerably. Migraine sufferers often find that cheese is a trigger. Soya milk and tofu (soya bean) products are now readily available in most health food shops and even some supermarkets – they are usually more acceptable to sensitive digestions.

8. If you snack between meals try to go for fruit, dried fruit and nuts, or raw vegetables rather than sweets or cakes. Some people need to work on the 'little and often' principle, especially if they tend to blood sugar swings. In this case a handful of almonds, sunflower seeds and raisins can be just as satisfying and in the long run better for health.

9. Finally, make sure that you drink a glass or two of plain water every day. The body needs a certain amount of water in order to carry on its necessary chemical processes; dehydration can result if this is not supplied. Water also helps to flush out toxins and so cleanse the body.

If you are changing your diet it is a good idea to introduce new measures slowly. There will be less chance of digestive problems or the family staging a mutiny when their favourite junk goes off the menu! I find that a whole food, vegetarian diet suits my system best as it provides plenty of energy and variety. As a Shiatsu practitioner I have a few personal rules, like not taking alcohol or very sweet food on days when I am practising or teaching. On the other hand I find that it does no harm to stray from the straight and narrow occasionally. There is nothing worse than someone whose diet is so restricted (by choice, not for medical reasons, I might add) that you can't take them out for a meal!

LIFESTYLE

Two other factors in good health which must not be forgotten are exercise and sleep. However fast a pace we live at or whatever our lifestyle, sleep and exercise are essential. Exercise we can place in two categories; aerobic, that is 'things that make you puff', like running, cycling, swimming, team games, racquet sports, even a brisk walk; and soft exercise which improves Ki circulation and flexibility, such as yoga, Tai Chi, Qi Gong, Do-In, and so on. I would suggest that everyone take a little of each kind; 20 minutes brisk exercise to stimulate the cardiovascular system three times per week, and 15 minutes soft exercise every day are good averages to aim for.

Sleep and rest are just as important. During the night our bodies rest and recuperate, building up our store of Ki for use the next day. Either too much sleep or too little can have a detrimental effect, but each of us must discover what routine works best. The gentle movements we make during sleeping hours allow us to relax and unknot our bodies subconsciously, while dreams may help us to work through the unfinished affairs of the day. Insomnia is a common problem for many people and in my experience it is the worry about not sleeping that is often more of a problem than the lack of sleep itself. If you find you waken at night and cannot get off to sleep again, *don't worry*. Although our bodies need sleep, they need rest just as much – tell yourself that although you are not sleeping, you *are* resting, and try some of the hara breathing exercises we looked at earlier in this chapter. After ten minutes or so of these you may find that your mind has quietened sufficiently to let you nod off again.

FIRST AID POINTS

Although a relaxing Shiatsu session may be just what we need when we are ill or in pain, sometimes it is not practicable. This is where we can make use of specific tsubo for first aid. Each practitioner has a list of useful points and those below are the ones I find most helpful in situations where a full session is not possible. Where you are using a tsubo as a remedy for a specific complaint, do remember that it is not a 'magic bullet' and results may not be immediate; for example if I use a point for a headache, I usually find that it takes about fifteen minutes of working the point on and off to produce a reduction in the pain. Press the point and get the sensation of connecting with Ki – generally a 'nice pain' or sensitivity. Hold that for between seven and ten seconds, then release for the same length of time. Continue on and off for a couple of minutes and then rest for a couple of minutes. If the point starts to feel very sensitive, try using another point with a similar action – points can often be used very effectively in combinations.

BL2: in the notch at the inside of the upper eye socket: frontal headache and sore eyes.

GB20: on the hollow between the two large neck muscles (trapezius and sternocleidomastoid) at the back of the neck, just under the skull: neck release point for tension and pain in the neck, one-sided headaches.

LU1: one thumbs-width below the hollow under the outside end of the collarbone: coughing, asthma, any lung problem.

LI10: three fingers-width down from the elbow crease, on top of the large forearm muscle: pain control in the arm and shoulders, intestinal problems.

LI4: in the fleshy web between thumb and index finger on the back of the hand and close to the bones: headache, toothache, brings Ki downwards in the body, constipation, diarrhoea, general toning of the intestines, helps to promote labour but forbidden in pregnancy.

HG6: two thumbs-width above the wrist crease on the inner arm, between the tendons: nausea and vomiting, especially morning sickness and sea sickness.

HG8: if you make a loose fist HG8 is where your middle finger touches the centre of your palm: for calming the mind if you are nervous or anxious.

HT7: at the wrist crease just inside the tendon on the little finger side: calms the mind, anxiety, insomnia, sweating at night, heart problems.

HT9: on the inside corner of the little finger nail: heart problems including heart attack (if other first-aid measures have been taken), severe anxiety.

GB30: in the centre of the buttock where there is a hollow when the muscle is clenched: sciatica, pain and tiredness in the legs, lower back pain.

ST36: four fingers-width below the outside bottom corner of the kneecap: indigestion, nausea and any stomach disorder, tiredness and pain in the legs, generally good for vitality.

SP6: three fingers-width up from the inner ankle starting the measurement from where the ankle begins to protrude (not from the highest part) just behind the bone: menstrual problems of any sort, especially menstrual pain, reproductive disorders, tiredness, relieves pain in the abdomen, calms the mind, insomnia. Avoid during pregnancy but useful in labour.

LV3: on the top of the foot in the hollow behind the second joint of the big toe, between first and second metatarsals: migraine, headaches, muscular cramps, calming effect especially on bad temper.

KD1: on the sole of the foot just below the ball in line with the second toe: tonifies the body's Yin energy, clears and calms the mind, can be used in cases of unconsciousness.

These points can be used safely on anyone, from children to the elderly. Use common sense, don't overstimulate, and if the condition persists seek advice from a qualified person.

MOXIBUSTION

Moxibustion is often used by Shiatsu practitioners in combination with Shiatsu to promote healing in cases where heat is beneficial. Processed from the common herb mugwort, Moxa is burnt either on or above specific tsubo in order to warm them, encourage local circulation and increase Ki flow into a point with a certain required action. Moxa punk looks rather like brown cotton wool. When used with the 'direct' method it is pinched into little cones which are then burnt down on a thin slice of ginger or garlic until the receiver feels a hot sensation. Rather more practical and less of a fiddle to use during a Shiatsu session is the 'indirect' method where the moxa punk has been compressed into a roll, rather like a long cigar, and this is held over the point, on and off, until it becomes reddish and feels pleasantly warm. Since moxa does not burn with a flame but merely smoulders, it is quite easy to regulate the heat by holding closer or further away, and the receiver is instructed to say when it becomes too hot. It goes without saying that the practitioner takes great care not to burn the skin. Treatment by moxa is very effective for cases of chronic pain, frozen shoulder, some kinds of arthritis, diarrhoea, coldness and general tiredness.

All of these adjuncts to treatment and exercises can be incorporated into our everyday lives when we start to take more responsibility for ourselves. By doing them we can feel and understand that by our own actions, activities and attitudes we can change our Ki state to one where we can become more in control and achieve what we want to in life.

7

Taking It Further

HOW TO FIND A PRACTITIONER

OVER THE PAST ten years complementary and alternative therapies have enjoyed a remarkable rise in popularity. Disillusionment with the drug-based treatment of orthodox medical practice coupled with a lack of time on the part of GPs and an increasing desire by patients to play a more active and responsible role in their own treatment have all, no doubt, played their part in turning a great many people towards gentler systems of medicine.

It is within the scope of most natural therapies to give each patient an understanding of their condition in relation to their overall health potential, and perhaps it is this quest for self understanding and the need for some sympathetic person with a different outlook and sufficient time to talk over health concerns that leads so many people into the realms of alternatives. However, once out of the established norms of orthodox medicine, there is the very real question of standards and qualifications. How to find a reputable practitioner? Is there a national regulatory organization? Is it best to approach a training school for their list of therapists? Do all schools train to the same standard? For the unfortunate patient who only wants someone to ease his back pain it can seem like a wilderness.

In Shiatsu we are very privileged to have an organization, the Shiatsu Society, which encompasses all practitioners, teachers, and students of Shiatsu, uniting anyone with an interest in Shiatsu and working to promote all aspects of the therapy from providing public information to setting standards of professional practice.

In 1981 a small group of teachers and students of Shiatsu met in London to discuss ways of forging links between those few pioneers involved in the therapy in Britain at that time.

From this initiative the Shiatsu Society was born. Originally conceived as a communications network, it soon took on the role of professional association and information point for the public, and published a register of practitioners. The setting of standards for professional training and practice was seen as the responsibility of the existing senior teachers and practitioners, resulting in discussions to set up in a system to unify standards while respecting each individual practitioner's unique way of working and taking into account the varying styles and philosophical approaches taught by different training establishments.

The Shiatsu Society therefore acts as an umbrella organization for Shiatsu in Britain. Ordinary membership is open to anyone with an interest in the therapy, whether a student of Shiatsu, someone from a medical or social work background, or a member of the public wanting to stay in contact. Practitioner and Teacher membership is extended to those who have fulfilled the Society's qualifying requirements.

One of the guiding ideals behind the Society has always been to encourage communication between practitioners and teachers of different styles and approaches to Shiatsu, in this way avoiding the disagreements which have dogged other therapies from time to time. All the major Shiatsu schools are run by Registered Teacher members of the Shiatsu Society, and graduates from the schools are eligible to sit the Society's practitioner assessment which governs entry to the *Register of Practitioners*. The Shiatsu Society's Register is a unified listing of practitioners from different training establishments who have completed a minimum of three years training, have passed their school's qualifying examinations, and have satisfied the Society's Assessment Panel of their professional competence in both practical and theoretical work. Registered Practitioners may use the designatory letters MRSS (Member of the Register of the Shiatsu Society). A full list of Registered Practitioners is available from:

The Shiatsu Society Administrator,
14 Oakdene Rd,
Redhill,
Surrey, RH1 6BT
Tel. 0737–767896.

113

As well as practitioners in Britain, the Society has several Registered Practitioners in Europe where not every country has a professional organization, and also maintains contacts with practitioners and therapy organizations internationally (see *contacts* section of this chapter, page 113).

TRAINING IN SHIATSU

Classes in Shiatsu are fairly widely available in this country, either as leisure interest evening classes at beginners level, or as professional training for those who wish to become practising therapists. Most classes are held on evenings or weekends, although one or two of the large colleges run day time professional courses. Although not yet as widespread as classes in, for example, yoga, teachers can be found from Brighton to Inverness, East Anglia to West Wales. Details of courses are available from the Shiatsu Society and are often advertized in the Society's quarterly newsletter.

Training in Shiatsu is not merely a question of learning the theory and techniques. As I have emphasized throughout this book, Shiatsu is about attitude, self-understanding and personal development. If you are serious in your intention to become a practitioner, I strongly suggest that you find a teacher or organization whom you feel you can trust and grow with – you may need to try several beginners classes before you find someone you really 'click' with.

Most schools do not have entrance requirements other than enthusiasm and motivation: many try to get away from the old academic ways of working which most of us had enough of at secondary school, so classes may include a large proportion of practical *hands-on* work, with *new games*, creative work, and sensitivity exercises included to facilitate learning with the whole body, the senses and the feelings as well as the mind. Of course, intellectual work is needed, especially at more advanced levels where oriental theory, diagnosis, anatomy, physiology and pathology form part of the curriculum. Some schools set practical and written homework, and some form of assessment is usually included at the end of a course.

Later in your training you will be encouraged to study with different teachers in order to broaden your outlook, increase your repertoire of techniques, and learn to respect other approaches to Shiatsu. Many schools run courses which take students up to Shiatsu Society Assessment standard; other individual teachers may offer classes in special aspects of Shiatsu or take pupils to certain levels before referring them on to other teachers.

The Shiatsu Society provides a list of Registered Teachers and recognized Shiatsu schools. The Society's quarterly newsletter also has details of classes being held throughout the country, as well as special seminars with teachers from abroad.

CONTACTS

Great Britain

The Shiatsu Society,
14 Oakdene Rd,
Redhill,
Surrey, RH1 6BT.
Tel. 0737–767896.

Eire

Shiatsu Society of Ireland
Greenville Lodge
Esker Road
Lucan
Co. Dublin

Europe

(consult The Shiatsu Society, Great Britain.)

USA

American Oriental Bodywork
   Therapy Association,
50 Maple Place,
Manhasset,
New York 11030, USA.

Japan

Japanese Shiatsu College,
2–15–6 Koishikawa,
Bunkyoku,
Tokyo,
Japan.

Iokai Centre,
1–8–9 Higashiuena,
Daito-Ku,
Tokyo,
Japan.

Australia

The Shiatsu Therapy Association of Australia,
332 Carlisle Street,
Balclava,
3183 Victoria
Australia.

In Conclusion

WHY SHIATSU?

I F WE LOOK on *healing* as the process of *becoming whole*, I firmly believe that each of us has the ability to heal others, in some way, if we choose to do so. I also believe that the desire to help and heal springs from our essential humanity and sympathy for the other living beings travelling with us on this complex, confusing, sometimes joyous and sometimes painful journey we call Life. How we choose to express our healing depends on us individually. Some of us bump into it early in life; others never manage to be tuned in sufficiently to be able to express this positive aspect of ourselves.

Personally, I fell into Shiatsu almost literally through practising the martial art Aikido. A fall on the mat and someone using tsubo to bring me round, a series of lectures on Yin Yang, and the development of ferocious migraine attacks all led me to investigate Shiatsu for the sake of my own health. I went on a weekend course and *that was it!* I had found what I wanted to do in life. Here was a way in which I could help others, in which I could communicate at a deep level – having taken a degree in languages and been involved in journalism prior to taking up Shiatsu, communication has always been important to me. At the same time I could work on my own health and personal strength. The discipline of Shiatsu practice appealed to me; also the fact that it harnesses one's power through the use of hara, yet uses this power in a compassionate and nurturing way. Its movement and creativity extended both my

116

body and mind, while my entry into the unseen world of the workings of Ki fascinated me. In short, Shiatsu as a medium for self expression and healing was completely aligned with my own energy quality. If I had been different I might have found another therapy, or spiritual healing, or yoga, or conventional medicine. There is a saying in esoteric teaching: 'When the pupil is ready the master will appear'; I feel that Shiatsu has been my master and teacher for many years guiding me to self understanding and a knowledge of my purpose in life.

I have no illusions that Shiatsu can cure all things; for me it is more a way of holding up a mirror and letting patients have a look at themselves. Sometimes this has the effect of helping them let go of pain or a longstanding health problem, or of helping them start to care for themselves. Sometimes Shiatsu helps someone get their life in order sufficiently to be able to cope with their troubles; sometimes it can help someone to die with dignity.

The power of compassionate touch is immense. The power of healing touch, used with a knowledge of energy in a system such as Shiatsu, has the ability to enhance people's lives in a tremendously positive way. By reaching out through Shiatsu and improving the quality of individual's lives we can perhaps improve the quality of Life for everyone upon our Earth.

Bibliography

Chaitow, L. *Soft Tissue Manipulation*, Thorsons, 1980.

Dawes, N. *The Shiatsu Workbook*, Piatkus, 1991.

Durckheim, K. von, *Hara: The Vital Centre of Man*, Unwin Paperbacks, 1962

Essentials of Chinese Acupuncture, Foreign Languages Press, Beijing, 1980.

Jarmey, C. and Tindall, J. *Acupressure for Common Ailments*, Gaia Books, 1991.

Jarmey, C. and Mojay, G. *Shiatsu: The Complete Guide*, Thorsons, 1991.

Kaptchuk, T. *Chinese Medicine: The Web that has No Weaver*, Rider, 1983.

Kushi, M. *How to see your Health*, Japan Publications, 1980.

Lao Tzu, *Tao Te Ching*, Penguin Classics, trans. Lau, 1963.

Lidell, L. *The Book of Massage*, Ebury Press, 1984.

Lundberg, P. *The Book of Shiatsu*, Gaia Books, 1992.

Maciocia, G. *The Foundations of Chinese Medicine*, Churchill Livingstone, 1989.

Masunaga, S. *Zen Imagery Exercises*, Japan Publications, 1987.

Masunaga, S. *Zen Shiatsu*, Japan Publications, 1977.

Namikoshi, T. *The Complete Book of Shiatsu Therapy*, Japan Publications, 1981.

Ohashi, W. *Do it Yourself Shiatsu*, Unwin Paperbacks, 1977.

Ploss & Bartels. *The Women*, Heineman (Medical), 1929.

Ridolfi, R. *Shiatsu*, Macdonald Optima, 1990.

Seem, M. *Bodymind Energetics*, Thorsons, 1988.

Serizawa, K. *Effective Tsubo Therapy*, Japan Publications, 1984.

Serizawa, K. *Tsubo: Vital Points for Oriental Therapy*, Japan Publications, 1976.

Suzuki, S. *Zen Mind, Beginners Mind*, Weatherhill, 1970.

Tohei, K. *Ki in Daily Life*, Japan Publications, 1978.

Veith, I. trans. *The Yellow Emperor's Classic of Internal Medicine*, University of California Press, 1966.

Yamamoto, S. *Barefoot Shiatsu*, Japan Publications, 1979.

Symptomatic Table of Meridians to use for Common Ailments

Symptoms	Relevant meridian to work
Colds/flu	Lung, & Triple Heater in the early stages
Headache (front head)	Bladder, Stomach
Headache (side head)	Gall Bladder & Liver
Headache (back head)	Bladder
Migraine	Liver (especially LV3) & Gall Bladder
Indigestion/nausea	Stomach, Spleen, Heart Governor (HG6)
Constipation/diarrhoea	Large Intestine & Small Intestine
Chestiness/coughing/asthma	Lung
Tiredness (chronic)	Kidney & Conception Vessel
Reproductive problems	Spleen, Liver & Kidneys
Back pain	Bladder, Governing Vessel & Gall Bladder
Sciatica	Gall Bladder & Bladder

If your partner is suffering from any of these common complaints, take a look back to the tables in Chapter 3 to see the theoretical connections and also consult the chart of common tsubo (page 109) to find out the best points to use on the relevant meridian. You can then work the whole of the meridian, paying particular attention to areas where Ki feels disturbed (generally the body will either feel tight and resisting or it will feel weak and empty), and to the classic points indicated for the problem.

Glossary

Acupressure: a system of healing similar to Shiatsu, but concentrating more on the classical points as used in Acupuncture.

Five Elements: (also translated as **Five Phases** or **Five Transformations.**) A theory used widely in oriental medicine in which energy is described by the elements Metal, Water, Wood, Fire and Earth. Encompasses a theory of energy flow between elements, and the grouping of similar phenomena into correspondences.

Hara: Japanese word for the abdomen, acknowledged as the centre of physical and spiritual strength; much used in Shiatsu to promote balance, sensitivity of touch and healing power.

Jing: the vital energy stored in the kidneys which regulates our pace of growth, maturity and ageing; also regulates our ability to reproduce.

Ki: Japanese word for energy, encompassing all phenomena in the universe, but used specifically in oriental medicine to describe the energy in the body.

Kyo-jitsu: the theory used in Zen Shiatsu to describe the way in which two meridians can be in a dynamic relationship where the empty or unresponsive (kyo) meridian is causing a full or over-reactive (jitsu) meridian to manifest elsewhere.

Meridian: a pathway of energy in the body where Ki flows more strongly. Each meridian is related to one of the internal organs and is therefore called after it.

Shen: the Spirit (also translated as Mind) referring to all the psychological and emotional elements to our individuality.

Shiatsu: Japanese word meaning 'finger pressure', used to describe a therapy which is rich in variety of technique and theory, and uses pressure with hands, thumbs, knees and feet to promote healing in the body, mind and spirit.

Tanden: a point three finger's width below the navel, at the centre of the **Hara.**

Tsubo: Japanese word for the classical points, usually to be found on meridians, although there are some non-meridian extraordinary points.

Yin-Yang: the dynamic underpinning all oriental medicine, in which complementary and opposite forces interact in a never ending flow: for example hot and cold, rising and falling, day and night, male and female.

Zen: a form of Buddhism which acknowledges that Enlightenment can occur at any time, encouraging spontaneity and living in the present; 'being here right now'.

Index